# FOODS
# THAT
# FIGHT
# CANCER

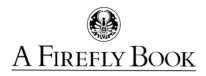

# A FIREFLY BOOK

Published by Firefly Books Ltd. 2016

Second printing

**Publisher Cataloging-in-Publication Data (U.S.)**

Names: Béliveau, Richard, 1953-, author. | Gingras, Denis, author. | Bruneau, Pierre, author. | Sandilands, Barbara, translator.
Title: Foods that fight cancer : preventing cancer through diet / authors, Richard Béliveau, Denis Gingras, Pierre Bruneau ; translated by Barbara Sandilands.
Description: Richmond Hill, Ontario, Canada : Firefly Books, 2016. | Includes bibliography and index | Originally published in French by Les Éditions du Trécarré, Quebec, Canada as Les aliments contre le Cancer | Summary: "This book will change the way you perceive cancer. It focuses on ways to fight and prevent the illness... It explains in detail phytochemicals, cancer-fighting molecule elements and which foods contain them... This science-based book explains the science behind each food recommendation and how it works" – Provided by publisher.
Identifiers: ISBN 978-1-77085-769-8 (paperback)
Subjects: Cancer – Nutritional aspects. | BISAC: HEALTH & FITNESS / Diseases / Cancer. | MEDICAL / Oncology.
Classification: LCC RC268.45B455 |DDC 616.9940654 – dc23

**Library and Archives Canada Cataloguing in Publication**

CIP data for this title is available from Library and Archives Canada

Published in the United States by
Firefly Books (U.S.) Inc.
P.O. Box 1338, Ellicott Station
Buffalo, New York 14205

Published in Canada by
Firefly Books Ltd.
50 Staples Avenue, Unit 1
Richmond Hill, Ontario L4B 0A7

Translated from French (Canada) by Barbara Sandilands

Printed in Canada

This book is dedicated to all those who are living with cancer.

Our sincerest thanks to the invaluable sponsors of the Chair in the Prevention and Treatment of Cancer, especially Nautilus Plus, whose financial support makes it possible for us to continue our research.

Developed by Les Éditions du Trécarré, Groupe Librex inc.,Une société de Québecor Média, La Tourelle, 1055, boul. René-Lévesque Est, Bureau 300, Montréal (Québec), H2L 4S5

For Groupe Librex: Editor **Miléna Stojanac**; Proofreader **Céline Bouchard et Julie Lalancette**; Interior design, and page layout: **Axel Pérez de León**; Illustrations: **Michel Rouleau;** Author photos: **Julien Faugère**

New, Revised Edition

# FOODS THAT FIGHT CANCER

## Preventing Cancer Through Diet

Richard Béliveau, PhD
& Denis Gingras, PhD
Translated by Barbara Sandilands

FIREFLY BOOKS

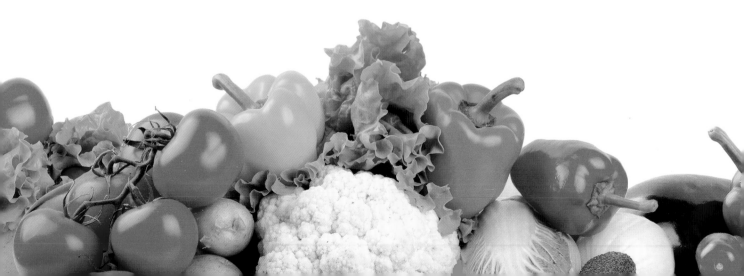

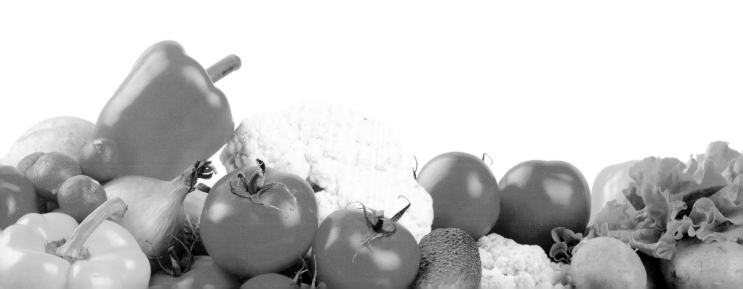

# Preface to the second edition

Our view of cancer has changed considerably in recent years. While cancer was long viewed as a devastating disease that appeared overnight, we now know that it is actually a chronic disease that in most cases takes several decades to reach a clinical stage. We all carry immature tumors inside us and are thus at high risk of developing cancer, but advances in research have clearly shown that it is possible to slow down the progression of these precancerous cells by adopting good lifestyle habits that will stop them from accumulating mutations and reaching a mature stage. The main objective in cancer prevention is therefore not so much to keep cancer cells from appearing, but rather to slow their progression down enough so that they cannot reach the mature cancer stage during the eight or nine decades of a human life.

In the last 10 years, several studies have confirmed that dietary habits in Western countries play a leading role in the high rate of cancer in our societies. Every country, without exception, that adopts the kind of diet fashionable in the West — high in sugar, meat and processed products, but low in plants — has to deal with an alarming increase in obesity, diabetes and several types of cancer.

The importance of these observations requires a complete update of this book to incorporate the latest research developments. The potential for cancer prevention remains absolutely remarkable, as two-thirds of all cancers can be avoided through simple changes in our lifestyle, including dietary habits.

# Preface to the first edition

Cancer continues to defy the progress made by modern medicine; after over 40 years of intensive research, it remains a mysterious killer, responsible for the premature deaths of millions of people each year. If some cancers are now treated with a good degree of success, many others are still very difficult to fight and represent a major cause of mortality among the active population. Now, more than ever, discovering new means of increasing the effectiveness of current anticancer therapies is of great importance.

The goal of this book is to present a summary of the scientific studies currently available. These studies strongly suggest that certain types of cancers can be prevented by modifying our dietary habits to include foods with the power to fight tumors at the source and thus prevent their growth. Nature supplies us with an abundance of foods rich in molecules with very powerful anticancer properties, capable of engaging with the disease without causing any harmful side effects. In many respects, these foods possess therapeutic properties on par with those of synthetic drugs; we propose calling them *nutraceuticals* to better illustrate these properties. We have the possibility of deploying a veritable arsenal of anticancer components occurring naturally in many foods as a complement to the therapies now in use. We can seize this occasion to change the probabilities in our favor, since a diet based on a regular intake of nutraceuticals may indeed prevent the appearance of many types of cancers.

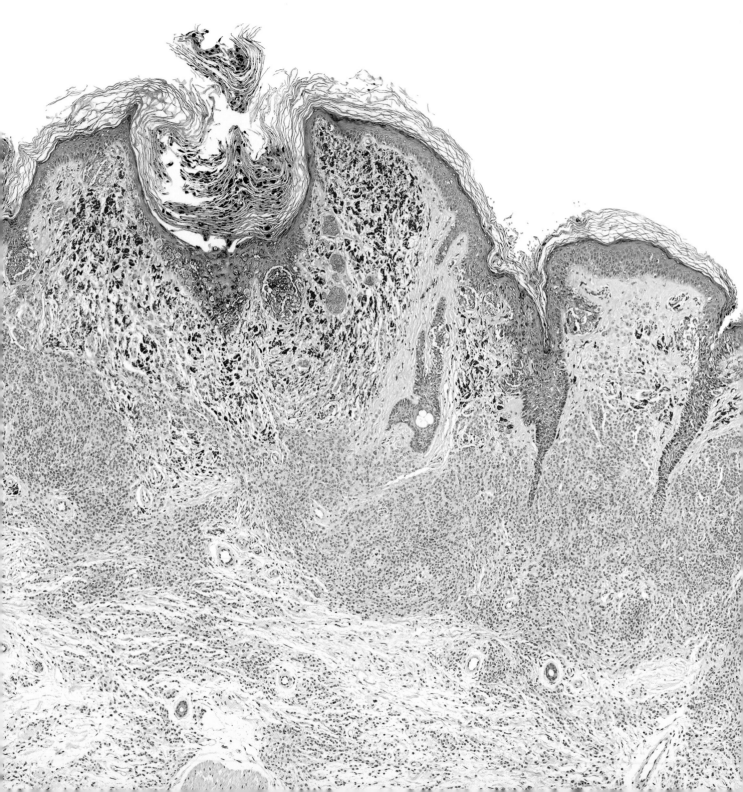

# Part I

# Cancer, a formidable enemy

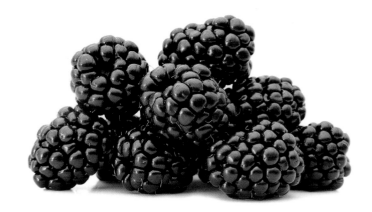

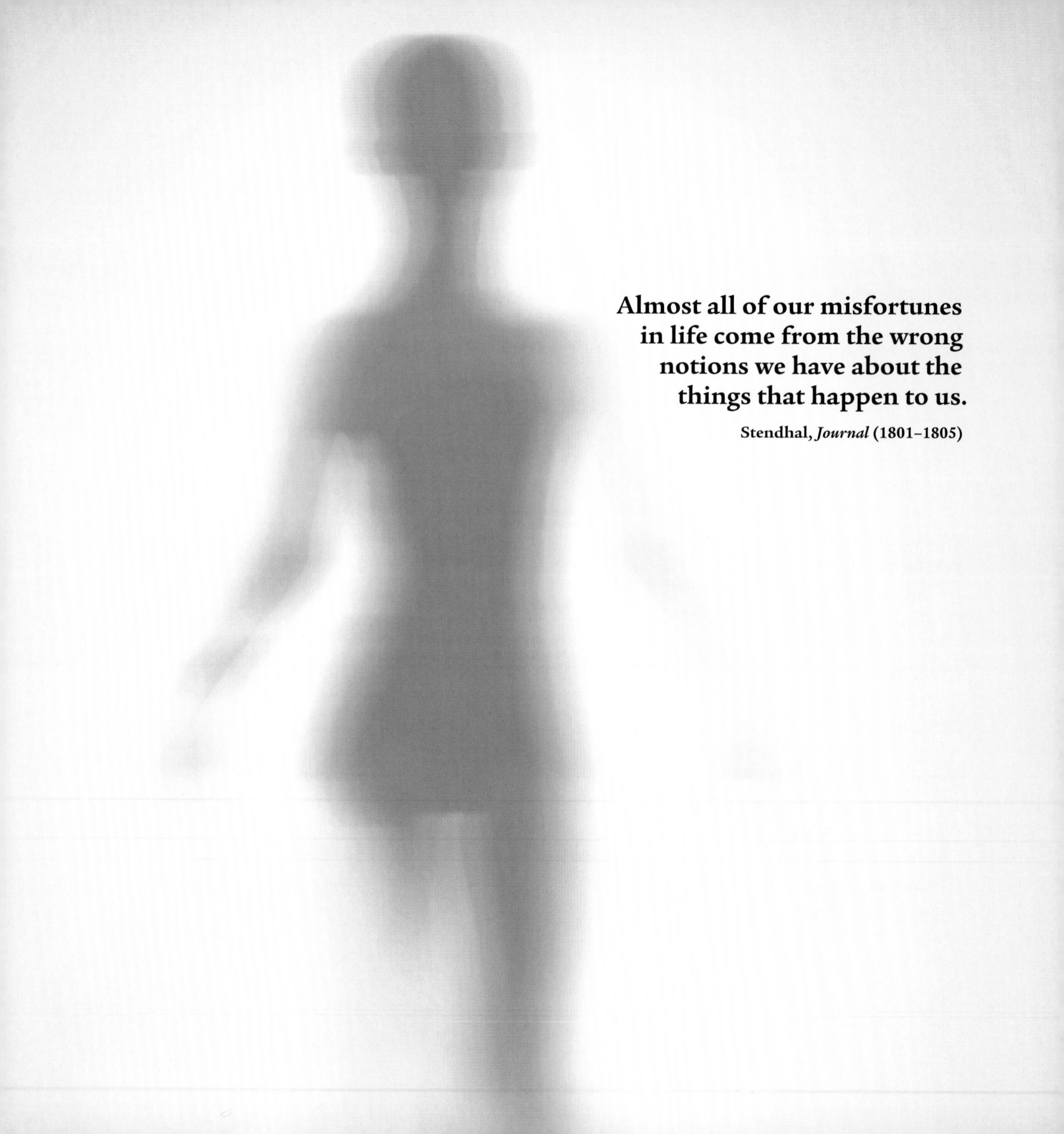

Almost all of our misfortunes
in life come from the wrong
notions we have about the
things that happen to us.

Stendhal, *Journal* (1801–1805)

# Chapter 1

# The Scourge of Cancer

## Cancer in figures

Some people are scared to death of flying, while others are terrified by sharks or lightning; the fear of harmful consequences that can result from events beyond our control seems to be a characteristic unique to the human species. Yet the actual risk of experiencing these extraordinary ordeals at some point is relatively slim compared with those risks directly related to daily life (Figure 1). For example, obese people are almost a million times more likely to die prematurely because of their excess weight than in an airplane crash, and any one of you is at least 50,000 times more likely to be struck by cancer than by lightning during your lifetime, and even more so if you adopt a risky behavior like smoking.

Among all of the real dangers we have to cope with, cancer is an undeniable threat: the disease will affect two out of five people before the age of 75, and one person in four will die from complications related to cancer. Every year, 10 million people around the world develop cancer and 7 million deaths are caused by the disease, amounting to 12 percent of all deaths recorded worldwide. And the situation is not getting any better, since it is now estimated that as the population gradually ages, 15 million new cancer cases will be diagnosed annually. In North America alone, 10 million people are currently living with cancer and 600,000 people will die of the disease in the coming year. To grasp the scope of the tragedy, imagine the TV news showing four Boeing 747s full of passengers crashing every day, or the collapse of the World Trade Center twin towers three times a week ... Not to mention the cost associated with treating people with cancer, evaluated at $180 billion annually, and which will only climb in coming years. These figures illustrate the size of the public health problem cancer poses and attest to the need to identify potential new ways to reduce the negative impacts of this disease on society.

Figures aside, cancer is first and foremost a human tragedy that takes away the people around us who are precious to us, deprives young children of their mother or father and leaves a wound that never heals in parents devastated by the loss of their child. The loss of loved ones causes an enormous feeling of injustice and anger, a sensation of being the victim of bad luck or of an unfortunate random attack we were not able to avoid. Not only does cancer take away human lives that are dear to us, but it also raises doubts about our ability to conquer it.

This feeling of powerlessness in the face of cancer is clearly reflected in public opinion surveys on the causes of the disease. Generally speaking, people view cancer as a disease triggered by uncontrollable factors: 89 percent of people think that cancer is caused by a genetic predisposition and more than 80 percent believe that environmental factors, like industrial pollution or pesticide residues on foods, are significant

| Our big fears ... and reality | |
|---|---|
| Fears | Actual risk |
| Dying in a shark attack | 1 in 252 million |
| Being struck by lightning | 1 in 1 million |
| Dying from food poisoning | 1 in 100,000 |
| Dying in a car accident | 1 in 7,000* |
| Getting food poisoning | 1 in 6 |
| Dying prematurely due to obesity | 1 in 5 |
| Getting heart disease | 1 in 4 |
| Getting cancer | 1 in 3 |
| Dying from the effects of smoking (smokers) | 1 in 2 |

* For people aged 25 to 34

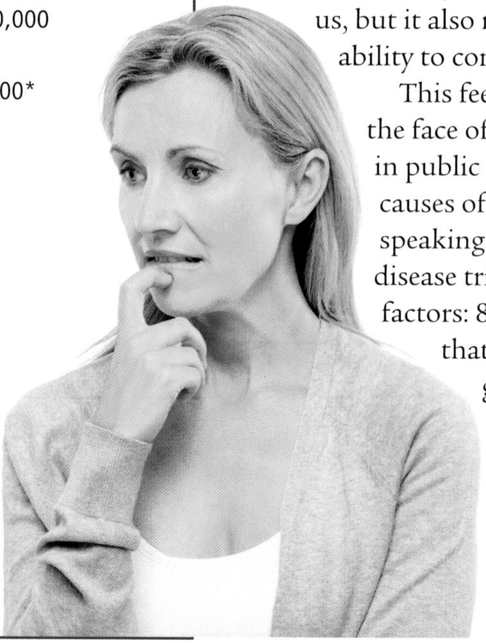

**Figure 1**          Adapted from *The Book of Odds*, 2013.

# Toning down heredity

The role of heredity in the development of cancer is much smaller than most people think. While there are indeed certain defective genes transmitted by heredity, increasing the risk of some cancers (BRCA genes, and breast and ovarian cancer, for example), these genes are very rare and all studies conducted to date clearly show that they do not play the critical role attributed to them. The comparison of cancer rates in identical and non-identical twins is a good example of this: if the risk of cancer were due to genes transmitted by heredity, identical twins with the same genes would be much more likely to both get the same disease than non-identical twins. This is not what has been observed for most cancers; when one twin got cancer during the study, fewer than 15 percent of identical twins developed the same cancer (Figure 2). Similarly, the simultaneous development of leukemia in identical twins is relatively rare: despite the presence of the same genetic anomalies in both children, only between 5 percent and 10 percent of pairs of twins get the disease at the same time.

The limited contribution of heredity to the development of cancer has also been clearly illustrated by the results of studies on children who were adopted very early in life. When one of the biological parents died of cancer before the age of 50, the risk of these children also getting the disease was increased by about 20 percent. On the other hand, when one of the adoptive parents died prematurely from cancer, a very large increase (500 percent) in cancer risk in these children was seen (Figure 3). In other words, the habits acquired while living with the adoptive parents (diet, physical exercise, smoking) had a far greater influence on cancer risk than the genes inherited from these children's biological parents.

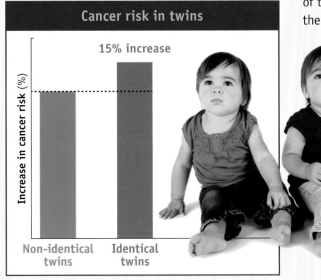

**Cancer risk in twins**

15% increase

Increase in cancer risk (%)

Non-identical twins    Identical twins

**Figure 2**          Adapted from Sørensen, 1988.

Even in cases where some defective genes are transmitted by heredity, it appears that cancer risk can be influenced greatly by lifestyle. For example, women carrying rare defective versions of the BRCA1 and BRCA2 genes have a breast cancer risk eight to 10 times higher than that of the general population and an ovarian cancer risk 40 times higher. However, the risk of developing early-onset breast cancer (before age 50) for women carrying these defective genes has tripled for those born after 1940 in comparison with those born before 1940, going from 24 percent to 67 percent. A determining role in this increased risk is attributed to the significant changes in lifestyle that have occurred since the Second World War (decreased physical activity, the industrialization of food, increased obesity). Overall, it is thought that the transmission of defective genes by heredity is responsible for roughly 15 percent to 20 percent of all cancers, meaning that most cancers are caused by external factors, probably related to lifestyle habits.

causes of cancer. In terms of lifestyle habits, an overwhelming majority of people (92 percent) associate smoking with cancer, but, conversely, less than half of people questioned think their diet can have an influence on the risk of developing the disease. Overall, these surveys show that people are rather pessimistic about their chances of preventing cancer, something not very likely or even impossible, according to half of them. Everyone concerned about public health should be worried about the results of these surveys and consider whether a thorough review of the communication strategies designed to inform the public about the causes of cancer is needed, since, with the exception of

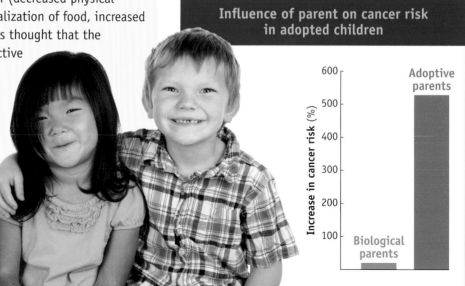

**Influence of parent on cancer risk in adopted children**

Increase in cancer risk (%)

Adoptive parents

Biological parents

**Figure 3**

Adapted by Sørensen, 1988.

smoking, these ideas run completely counter to what research has succeeded in identifying as triggering factors for cancer.

## A world map of cancer

This influence of lifestyle on cancer development is dramatically illustrated by examining the distribution of cancer cases worldwide (Figure 4). The cancer burden is not evenly distributed around the world. According to the latest statistics published by the World Health Organization, industrialized Western regions like North America, Australia and

several countries in Europe are the hardest hit by cancer, with more than 250 cases for every 100,000 inhabitants. In contrast, Asian countries like India, China and Thailand have much lower rates of cancer, with approximately 100 cases per 100,000 people.

Not only is the cancer burden distributed unequally from one region of the world to another, but, in addition, the types of cancer occurring in the populations of these different countries vary widely. Generally speaking, aside from lung cancer — the most common and most evenly widespread cancer worldwide (because of smoking) — the most common cancers in Western industrialized countries,

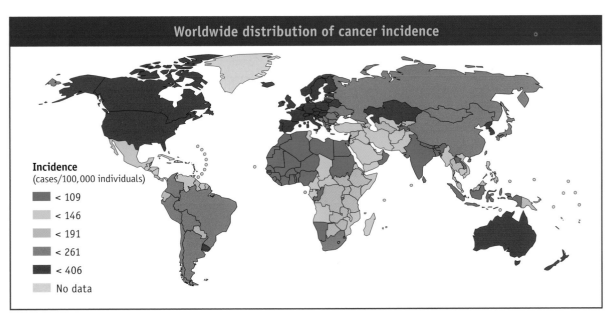

**Figure 4**

Source: GLOBOCAN 2004 (IARC).

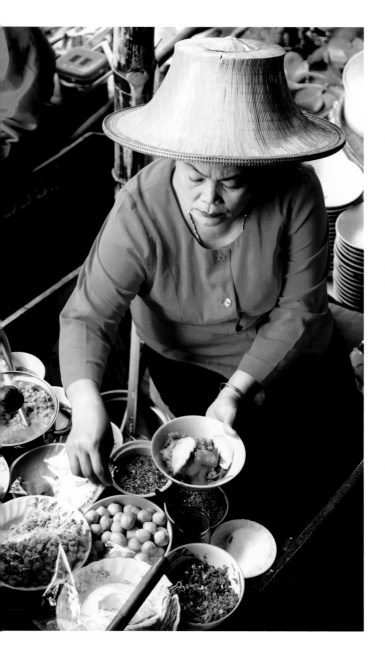

like the United States, are completely different from those occurring in Asian countries. In the United States and Canada, in addition to lung cancer, the main cancers are, in order, colon, breast and prostate cancer, while in Asian countries the incidence of these cancers is far lower than that of stomach, esophageal and liver cancer. The size of these differences between East and West is striking: for example, in some parts of the United States, more than 100 women in 100,000 get breast cancer, compared with just eight Thai women in 100,000. The same is true for colon cancer: whereas in some regions in the West, 50 people out of every 100,000 develop this cancer, it occurs in just five out of every 100,000 people in India. As for prostate cancer, the other major cancer in Western countries, the gap is even larger: it affects 10 times fewer Japanese men and as many as 100 times fewer Thai men than it does men in Western countries.

The study of migrant populations has made it possible to confirm that these extreme variations are not the result of some kind of genetic predisposition, but are instead closely related to differences in lifestyle. Figure 5 shows a striking example of the variations caused by immigration. In this study, figures on cancer incidence among Japanese living in Japan and those who had immigrated to Hawaii were compared with figures for the native-born Hawaiian population. For example, whereas prostate cancer was, at the time of the study, not very common in Japan, the incidence of this cancer increased tenfold among Japanese immigrants, to the point where it was almost the same as for native-born Hawaiians. The situation was similar for Japanese women, whose low rates of breast and uterine cancer increased considerably when they changed their lifestyle by emigrating.

These statistics do not represent an isolated case; far from it, as similar results have been obtained by studying various world populations. We will mention just one other example, a comparison of the incidence of certain types of cancer in the African-American population and in an African population in Nigeria (Figure 6). Once again, the Africans have cancer rates that are dramatically different from those among

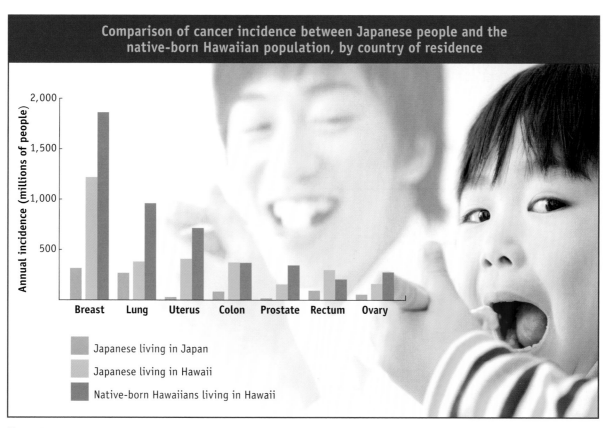

Comparison of cancer incidence between Japanese people and the native-born Hawaiian population, by country of residence

Annual incidence (millions of people)

Breast   Lung   Uterus   Colon   Prostate   Rectum   Ovary

■ Japanese living in Japan
■ Japanese living in Hawaii
■ Native-born Hawaiians living in Hawaii

**Figure 5**

Adapted from Doll and Peto, 1981.

African-Americans: the rate of prostate cancer is much higher in the United States than in Africa. In every case, the incidence of cancers in the African-American population studied is almost identical to that of Caucasian-Americans, while it is completely different from that of the African population in Nigeria. These studies are extremely interesting, since, in addition to providing irrefutable proof that most cancers are not the result of hereditary factors, they highlight the predominant role played by lifestyle in the development of the disease.

But what change can have had such a negative influence on the health of these emigrants as to result so quickly in an increase in cancer rate? All studies done up until now point to emigrants' rejection of their traditional diet and their rapid adaptation to the culinary traditions of the host country. In the two cases that interest us, these changes are tragic:

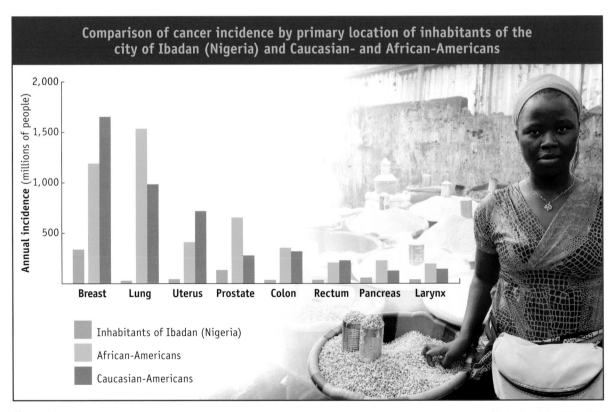

**Comparison of cancer incidence by primary location of inhabitants of the city of Ibadan (Nigeria) and Caucasian- and African-Americans**

Inhabitants of Ibadan (Nigeria)

African-Americans

Caucasian-Americans

**Figure 6**

Adapted from Doll and Peto, 1981.

18

for example, Japanese migrating to the West traded an exemplary diet, high in complex carbohydrates and vegetables, and low in fats, for a diet high in sugar, protein and animal fats.

Furthermore, quite aside from emigration, Japanese dietary habits have undergone major upheavals during the last 50 years that also illustrate the role of diet in cancer development. For example, whereas barely 40 years ago meat consumption was very rare in Japan, it has risen more than seven times in recent years, increasing the colon cancer rate fivefold to equal that of Western countries. It is alarming to realize the degree to which adopting a Western lifestyle has very clearly increased the incidence of a number of cancers.

## The real causes of cancer

Taken all together, these observations thus indicate that only a minority of cancers are caused by factors that really are beyond our control, such as heredity, environmental pollution or viral infections (Figure 7). Conversely, studies conducted by all cancer organizations, including the American Association for Cancer Research (AACR), show that several factors directly related to people's lifestyles, like smoking, physical inactivity, obesity, composition of the diet and the immoderate use of alcohol and narcotics, are

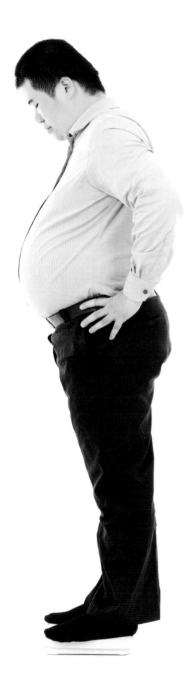

direct causes of the development of about 70 percent of cancers.

Re-examining our misconceptions about the causes of cancer is important, since it motivates us to change our defeatist approach to the disease and tackle the problem from a new angle. If two-thirds of cancers are caused by factors other than our genes and are instead related to our lifestyle habits, does this not therefore imply that we can avoid two out of three cancers by changing this lifestyle?

This is precisely the conclusion reached by scientists who have examined hundreds of thousands of studies on the impact of lifestyle habits on the risk of getting cancer. Thanks to these rigorous analyses carried out by cancer organizations worldwide, such as the World Cancer Research Fund, the American Cancer Society and the Canadian Cancer Society, it is possible to identify 10 key aspects of lifestyle that increase cancer risk and to adopt, as a result, certain behaviors that neutralize this

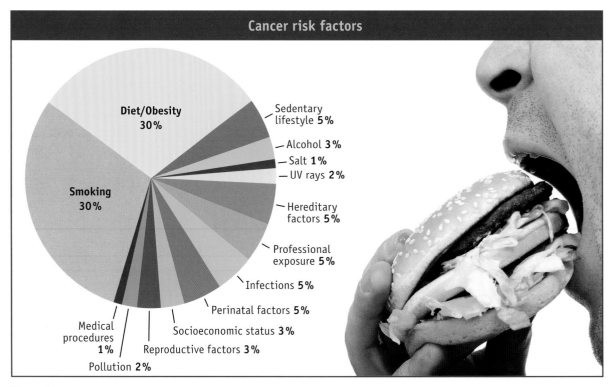

**Cancer risk factors**

Diet/Obesity 30%
Smoking 30%
Sedentary lifestyle 5%
Alcohol 3%
Salt 1%
UV rays 2%
Hereditary factors 5%
Professional exposure 5%
Infections 5%
Perinatal factors 5%
Socioeconomic status 3%
Reproductive factors 3%
Pollution 2%
Medical procedures 1%

**Figure 7**

Adapted from *AACR Cancer Progress Report*, 2011.

| | Risk factors | | Recommendations from cancer organizations |
|---|---|---|---|
| **Carcinogenic agents** | Smoking | | Stop smoking. |
| | Too much alcohol | | Limit daily alcohol consumption to two glasses for men and one for women. |
| | Excessive exposure to UV rays | | Protect the skin from the sun by avoiding unnecessary sun exposure. Avoid exposure to artificial sources of UV rays (tanning beds). |
| **Diet and control of body weight** | Sedentary lifestyle | | Be physically active at least 30 minutes every day. |
| | Lack of plant-based foods | | Eat more of a wide variety of fruits, vegetables and legumes, as well as foods based on whole grains. |
| | Excess weight and obesity | | Stay as lean as possible, with a body mass index of between 21 and 23. |
| | Processed foods (junk food) | | Avoid carbonated beverages and limit as much as possible the consumption of energy-dense foods containing large amounts of sugar and fat. |
| | Too much red meat and processed meats | | Limit the consumption of red meat (beef, lamb, pork) to approximately 18 ounces/500 g per week, replacing it with meals based on fish, eggs or vegetable proteins. Limit processed meats to a minimum. |
| | Too much salt | | Limit consumption of products preserved with salt (salt fish, for example), as well as products containing large amounts of salt. |
| | Taking supplements | | Don't make up for a bad diet by taking supplements: the synergy provided by a combination of foods is by far superior for lowering the risk of cancer. |

**Recommendations**

Figure 8

risk and could therefore significantly reduce the incidence of cancer in our societies (Figure 8). A crucial aspect, generally well-known to most people, is of course to reduce to a minimum exposure to cancer-causing agents like cigarette smoke, alcohol and ultraviolet rays. Tobacco alone is responsible for a third of all cancers, owing to the dramatic increase in risk of lung cancer and 15 or so other types of cancer in smokers, whereas alcohol and UV rays are well-characterized inducing agents for cancers of the digestive system and skin, respectively.

What is less well-known is the degree to which poor dietary habits and excess body weight can also be important factors for cancer risk. A lack of plant foods, and eating too many foods high in sugar and fat, too much red meat and processed meats, as well as foods high in salt, have all been associated with a higher risk of cancer, just like excess body weight and physical inactivity. Altogether, it is thought that the aspects of lifestyle related to diet and weight are responsible for roughly a third of all cancers, a percentage as high as that caused by tobacco, the most significant cancer-causing agent described to date (Figure 7). The proportion of deaths from cancer directly linked to the modern diet could actually be as high as 70 percent in the case of cancers of the gastrointestinal system (esophagus, stomach and colon). The foods we eat daily thus have an enormous influence on our risk of getting cancer, and current dietary habits absolutely must be changed if we want to reduce the burden cancer imposes on our society.

## The impact of diet on cancer

To try to understand how the nature of diet can contribute to this extent to the development of cancer, we must first understand just how unbalanced the modern diet is, both in its excesses and its deficiencies. In the West, the act of eating is often viewed simply as a way to supply the body with the energy essential for its survival; this viewpoint translates into a diet centered mainly on calorie consumption, with foods low in energy density like fruits and vegetables playing only a limited role. This tendency is exacerbated by the avalanche of processed foods overloaded with sugar and fat that are everywhere in our environment, encouraging us to eat too much and leading to an excessive accumulation of body fat. The modern Western diet has nothing to do with what was the very essence of the human diet barely 10 generations ago: today's diet contains at least twice the amount of fats, a percentage of saturated fat much higher in comparison with unsaturated fats, barely a third of the fiber intake, a flood of simple sugars to the detriment of complex carbohydrates and, paradoxically, a decrease in essential elements found in plants.

This kind of diet represents the worst possible combination for maintaining health and the best for encouraging cancer development. On the one hand, the excess calories lead to an increase in body weight, and many studies have clearly shown that excess weight and obesity are associated with increased risk for several types of cancer. On the other, low consumption of plant products deprives the body of several thousand anti-inflammatory and anticancer molecules that can hinder the progression of cancer cells and reduce the incidence of several types of cancer (Figure 9).

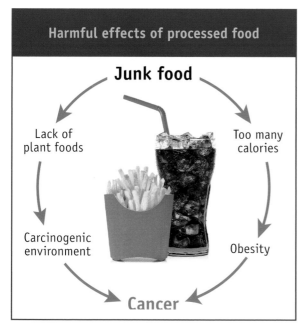

**Figure 9**

Furthermore, we are now seeing in real time the negative impact of this kind of diet worldwide. Every country that has changed its dietary traditions to incorporate those in fashion in North America also sees a rapid increase in its rates of obesity, colon and prostate cancer and heart disease – all diseases that for them were relatively rare in the past.

This kind of diet must therefore be called into question, not just for its excesses, monotony and lack of originality, but especially for its extremely negative impact on health. Nowadays, we accept with remarkable passivity the barrage of promotional advertising for fast food combos consisting of gigantic hamburgers, fries and oversized soft drinks, potato chips stuffed with "trans" fat and acrylamide, and other "snacks" constantly advertised on prime-time TV. Accepting the promotion of this kind of diet means we are resigning ourselves to spending large amounts of money on taking care of the health problems of future generations.

A significant change in this diet is an overriding objective in any prevention strategy designed to reduce the number of cancers occurring in the Western population. Fortunately, more and more people want to change their food habits, and they can rely on an ever-increasing number of products of excellent quality, made from healthy ingredients that really can contribute to better overall health. The vast majority of supermarkets now have a section where these foods are prominently displayed, not to mention the countless markets where we can become familiar with ingredients typical of cuisines from around the world that were, for the most part, unknown to us a mere 30 years ago. Indeed, while globalization has harmful effects for people who adopt a Western way of life, people in Western countries, on the other hand, benefit from the spread of culinary traditions from other cultures. There is most definitely an alternative to Western junk food for those who want to eat a healthy diet and protect themselves against serious diseases like cancer.

The purpose of this book is not to propose a diet. There are excellent books that have described the basic principles of a healthy diet, where you can find all pertinent information on how to achieve a balanced intake of proteins, fats and sugars, as well as vitamins and minerals. Instead, we hope to introduce you to a few foods that can genuinely help decrease the risk of developing this disease. These recommendations are obviously based on the well-established role of plant foods as a fundamental component of any diet designed to fight cancer, but they also take into account new scientific data suggesting that the *kinds* of fruits and vegetables consumed might play as important a role as the *amount*, since some foods are particularly good sources of anticancer molecules. It is therefore not just a question of eating the minimum of five servings of fruits and vegetables — we have to deliberately choose those most able to prevent the development of cancer. A diet based on an intake of foods high in anticancer compounds is an indispensable weapon for warding off cancer.

**In summary:**

- People's lifestyles play a predominant role in the risk of developing cancer.

- Approximately one-third of cancers are directly linked to diet.

- A diversified diet, high in fruits and vegetables, in tandem with controlled calorie intake so as to avoid becoming overweight, is a simple and effective way to significantly reduce the risk of getting cancer.

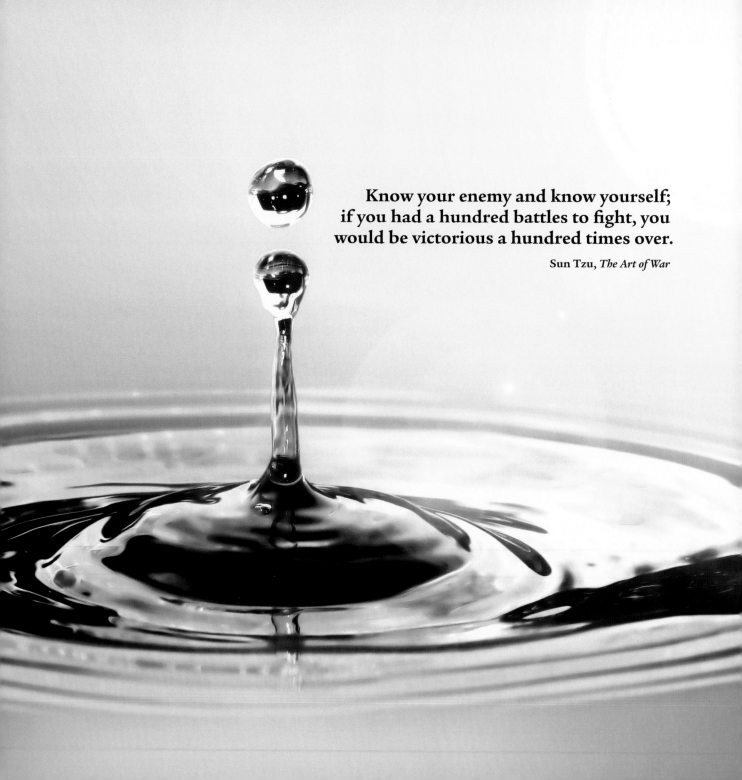

Know your enemy and know yourself;
if you had a hundred battles to fight, you
would be victorious a hundred times over.

Sun Tzu, *The Art of War*

# Chapter 2

# What Is Cancer?

Despite decades of painstaking research to the tune of billions of dollars, a great many cancers remain impossible to treat, and even when treatments are available for some types of cancer, patients' long-term survival often still falls short of expectations. Often, new drugs arousing much enthusiasm prove to be less effective than predicted, and even, in some cases, totally ineffective. What makes cancer so difficult to treat? This is a key question we need to consider before discussing new methods by which we can hope to fight this disease.

To use the people around us as an analogy, it is often possible to get to know the broad outlines of the character, motivations, strengths and weaknesses of an individual without necessarily having to learn all the details of his or her life. This is really what this chapter is all about: getting to know a cancer cell by looking only at the broad outlines of its "personality," at the motivations that cause it to invade surrounding tissues and grow to the point where it threatens a person's life; discovering how it is allowed to do this; and, even more importantly, identifying its weaknesses so as to better defend against it. Understanding what cancer is makes us realize just how fearsome an enemy cancer can be and how we must approach it with the greatest respect to avoid attack. But most importantly, by understanding what cancer is, we learn to exploit its weaknesses and keep it at bay.

## The root of all evil: The cell

The cell is the unit at the base of everything living on Earth, from the most humble bacterium with just one cell, to complex organisms like human beings, which contain over 37,000 billion. This tiny structure measuring barely 10–100 *µm* (a *µm* is one-thousandth of a millimeter) is truly a masterpiece of nature, a puzzle of unheard-of complexity that continues to astonish scientists trying to unravel its secrets. The cell is far from having revealed all of its secrets, but we already know that it is the disruption of some of its functions that plays a key role in cancer development. From a scientific point of view, cancer is first and foremost a cell disease.

To better understand the cell, we can compare it to a city where all of the functions essential to the community have been divided among different locations, so that workers can have optimal conditions in which to do their work. In terms of cancer development, four main components of the cell play an important role (Figure 10).

### The nucleus
This is the cell's library, the place where all the legal texts governing the city's functioning — *the genes* — are stored. The cells contain about 25,000 laws located inside a thick text, the DNA, which is written in a strange alphabet made up of just four letters: A, T, C and G. Reading these laws is important, for this tells the cell how to behave by causing it to produce the *proteins* it needs to function properly and respond to all of the changes occurring in its environment. For example, a warning signaling that the cell is running out of sugar will immediately be followed by the reading of a law authorizing the production of new proteins specialized for transporting sugar; the result is the replenishing of sufficient reserves so the cell can survive. When errors occur in reading these laws, the proteins formed are incapable of correctly carrying out their function and may thus contribute to the development of cancer.

### The proteins
The proteins are the city's "workforce," the molecules that carry out most of the functions necessary to maintain the cell's cohesion: transporting nutritive substances from the bloodstream, communicating messages from outside to inform the cell of changes in the external world, transforming nutrients to produce energy, etc. Several proteins are *enzymes*, the engineers of the cell, with the ability to transform unusable substances into proteins essential for the life of the cell. A number of enzymes also enable the cell to adapt quickly to any change in the environment by subtly modifying the functioning of other proteins. This means that the cell has to constantly make

sure that the reading of the laws governing the production of these enzymes is true to the original text, since an incorrect reading causes the production of modified proteins that are no longer able to accomplish their work correctly or whose overzealousness is not compatible with the cell's proper balance. Cancer is thus always caused by errors in protein production, especially enzymes.

### The mitochondria

This is the city's power station, the place where energy contained in the structure of molecules supplied by food (sugars, proteins and fats) is converted into cellular energy (ATP). Oxygen is used as fuel for this function, which, however,

causes toxic waste products called free radicals to form. These waste products can act as triggering elements for cancer by introducing changes into the law texts (genes) — mutations resulting in errors in protein production.

### The plasma membrane

This structure, which surrounds the cell, is made up of fats and certain proteins and acts as a wall to contain all of the cell's activities in one place. The plasma membrane plays a very important role, as it acts as a barrier between the interior of the cell and the external environment, a kind of filter that determines which substances can enter the cell and which can leave. It contains several proteins,

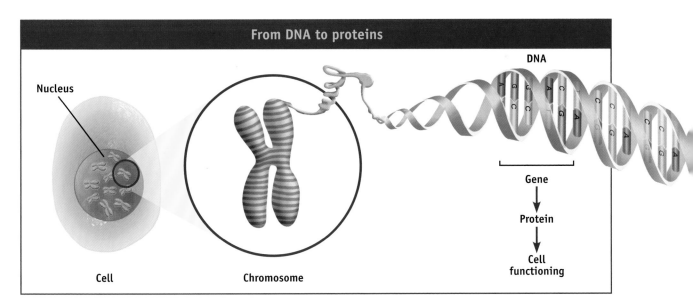

**From DNA to proteins**

Nucleus

DNA

Cell

Chromosome

Gene

Protein

Cell functioning

**Figure 10**

called receptors, that detect chemical signals in the bloodstream and transmit to the cell the coded messages sent by these signals in order to enable it to react to variations in its environment. This function is critical for the cell; obviously, an incorrect reading of the genes controlling protein production may have tragic consequences. When a cell can no longer understand what is happening outside, it loses its points of reference and begins to behave autonomously without regard for the other cells around it — very dangerous behavior that can lead to cancer.

## The constraints of communal living

What makes a cell become cancerous? Most people know that cancer is the result of the excessive cell multiplication, but in general the reasons that trigger this kind of behavior remain mysterious. Just as with any modern-day psychological analysis, the answer lies in the cell's childhood.

Today's cell is the result of the evolution of a primitive cell that appeared on Earth roughly 3.5 billion years ago, which resembled a bacterium much more than it did the cell we know today. During this long period, this ancestral cell was subjected to enormous variations in its environment (e.g., UV rays, oxygen levels) that forced it to continually search through trial and error for the modification that would give it the best chance of survival. The cell's great adaptability is due to its ability to modify its genes so as to produce new, more effective proteins to cope with new difficulties. It must be understood that the genes in cells, those so-called "laws" previously mentioned, are not unchanging. As soon as the cell senses that it would be a good idea to modify its laws to overcome a difficulty, it changes the text in the hope of doing so; this is what we call a mutation. Cells' ability to cause their genes to mutate is therefore an essential characteristic of life, without which we would never have existed.

Approximately 600 million years ago, cells made the "decision" that in the entire history of evolution would have the greatest consequences for the nature of life on Earth: they began to come together to form the first multicellular organisms. This was a radical change in the cell's "mindset," for cohabitation assumed that the organism's survival as a whole was more important than that of individual cells. This meant that the constant search for improvements to adapt to environmental changes could no longer continue to the detriment of the organism's other cells. In other words, from being individualistic, cells gradually became altruistic, and, in a way, gave up their fundamental freedom to change their genes as they wanted. This evolution was retained, since it provided considerable advantages, the most important being that the various cells could divide up the tasks so as to better interact with the environment. For example, in primitive organisms some cells became expert in the tasks associated with identifying nutrients in their immediate environment, whereas others instead became specialized in digesting foods to supply the organism with energy. To arrive at this specialization, cells changed their laws to create new kinds of proteins that improved their performance and enabled them to accomplish their tasks even more efficiently. The ability to adapt is at the heart of evolution, but, in the case of multicellular organisms, this adaptation absolutely has to benefit all of the cells in the organism.

In human beings, cell specialization has reached the heights of complexity. In fact, it is hard to believe that a skin cell, for example, is in any way related to a kidney cell. Or that muscle cells share a common origin with the neurons that allow us to think. Yet all cells in the human body contain in their nucleus the *same* genetic baggage, the same legal codebooks. A skin cell is different from a kidney cell not because the two kinds of cell do not have the same genes, but rather because they do not *use* the same genes to carry out their functions. In other words, each cell in the human body uses only those genes that correspond to its function; this is called cell differentiation. Maintaining cell differentiation is crucial for the body's proper functioning; if the neurons that allow us to think suddenly decided to behave like skin cells and no longer transmit any nerve impulses, the entire body would suffer. The same is true for all of our organs; each kind of cell must perform the task assigned to it for the well-being of the cells as a whole (the organism). When we consider that the human body contains 37,200 billion cells, each listening to the others, we cannot help but be astonished by the order that emerges out of such complexity.

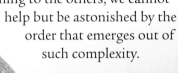

## Civil disobedience

Given that the proper functioning of an organism as complex as a human being requires the total repression of cells' ancestral survival instincts, as well as the sharing of all of their resources, it is easy to see that maintaining these functions is a delicate balancing act, constantly subject to attempts at "rebellion" by cells that want to reclaim their freedom of action. This is exactly what happens throughout our lifetime: as soon as a cell is attacked from the outside, whether by a cancer-causing substance, a virus or perhaps a surplus of free radicals, its first reflex is to interpret this attack as a test it must confront as best it can by mutating its genes to overcome this obstacle. These attacks occur frequently during our lifetime, with the result that many damaged cells rebel and in so doing forget their primary function in the organism as a whole. Fortunately, to prevent the damaged cell from becoming too autonomous, the "good will" of cells is strictly governed by rules that ensure that social behavior is always respected; this allows rebel cells to be quickly eliminated and ensures that vital functions are maintained.

However, the application of these rules is not perfect; some cells still manage to find gene mutations that allow them to overcome these regulations and cause cancer.

**Rule 1**
Reproduction is not permitted, except to replace a damaged or dead cell.

**Rule 2**
Staying alive is not permitted if the cell structure is found to be damaged, especially the DNA. If the damage is too great, suicide is essential!

In other words, cancer appears when a cell stops being resigned to playing the role assigned to it and no longer agrees to cooperate with the others to dedicate its resources to the benefit of all the other calls in the organism. This cell becomes an outlaw isolating itself from its fellows and no longer responding to orders from the society in which it lives. Henceforth, it has only one thing on its mind: ensuring its own survival and that of its descendants. At this point, anything can happen: the rebel cell has rediscovered its ancestral survival instincts.

## The development of cancer

It is important to understand that cell transformation does not in itself mean that a cancer will immediately develop in the organism. As we will see later on, this delinquent behavior in cells occurs regularly during the life of an individual, without necessarily degenerating into cancer. Instead, cancer development must be seen as a gradual process that can occur quietly over several years or even several decades, before causing symptoms to appear. Cancer's "slowness" to develop is extremely important for us, since, as we will see throughout this book, it gives us a golden opportunity to intervene at several stages in its development and to block the evolution of a transformed cell into a mature cancer cell. Although every cancer has its own triggering factors, all cancers follow substantially the same development process, divided into three main stages: initiation, promotion and progression (Figure 11).

## 1. Initiation

Initiation is, as its name indicates, the initial stage in the cancer process, during which the first mutation appears in cell DNA. These mutations can be caused by exposure to a carcinogenic agent (ultraviolet rays, cigarette smoke, some viruses), by errors that occur spontaneously in genes during cell renewal or by genetic defects passed on through heredity.

With a few exceptions (some pediatric cancers, for example), the "initiated" cells are not yet sufficiently activated at this stage to be deemed cancerous; rather, they have the *potential* to form tumors if exposure to toxic agents continues to occur regularly or if a promotion factor allows the initiated cell to keep trying to find new mutations to

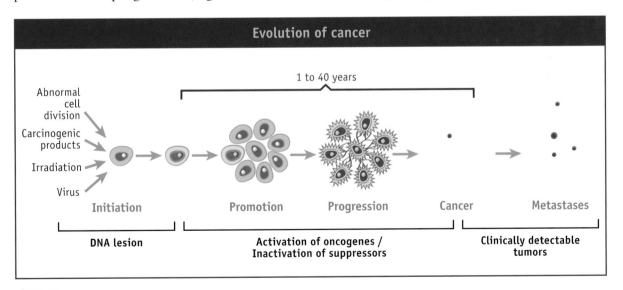

Figure 11

help it develop autonomously. As we will see, certain molecules in food have the property of maintaining these potential tumors in a latent state and can thus prevent cancer from developing.

### 2. Promotion

During this stage, the initiated cell overcomes rules 1 and 2 mentioned previously and reaches the critical threshold for becoming a transformed cell. The vast majority of current cancer research focuses on identifying the factors that allow the cell to overcome these two rules. In general, to disobey Rule 1 successfully, cancer cells release large amounts of proteins that enable cells to grow autonomously, without outside help. At the same time, a cell that is trying to become cancerous must eliminate the proteins responsible for applying Rule 2, without which all its efforts will be immediately countered by a cell suicide mechanism called *apoptosis* (see box). In both cases, mutations causing a change in protein function will result in the uncontrolled growth of modified cells and make them immortal. This is, however, a difficult stage that extends over a long period of time (from one to 40 years), since the cell has to make many attempts at mutation in the hope of acquiring the characteristics needed for its growth (Figure 11). The factors that encourage disobedience to the two major rules governing the life of the cell are still poorly understood,

but it is possible that certain hormones and growth factors, as well as the levels of free radicals, all play a role in this crucial stage. Nonetheless, it is a fairly safe assumption that the promotion phase is the one offering the best opportunity to intervene in the prevention of cancer development, since several of the factors involved can be largely controlled by individuals' lifestyles. As we will see in detail in the following chapter, several diet-related factors can influence this stage positively by forcing the future tumor to remain in this early stage. This prevention is crucial, for transformed cells that have succeeded in passing through the first two stages are extremely dangerous and will become even more so during the progression stage.

## The suicidal instincts of cells

Cells have developed an extremely detailed and aggressive program to force damaged or no longer functioning cells into retirement: suicide! Through apoptosis, the organism is able to "cleanly" destroy a cell without causing damage to neighboring cells and without causing inflammatory reactions in the tissues. Apoptosis is thus a vital aspect of several physiological processes, such as embryonic development, the elimination of ineffective immune cells and, a trouble spot for cancer, the destruction of cells displaying significant DNA damage.

*3. Progression*

It is really during this process that the transformed cell gains its independence and a growing number of malignant traits enable it to invade the surrounding tissue and even to spread into other tissues in the organism as metastases. All cancer cells in tumors that have succeeded in reaching this stage have six common characteristics, considered to be the "hallmarks" of a mature cancer (see box). This is why cancer is such a hard disease to treat: by acquiring all of these new properties, cancer cells that have reached maturity have in a way become a new life form able to replicate itself autonomously and resist a whole range of unfavorable conditions.

## Treating cancer: The limits of current approaches

There is no universal procedure used to treat cancer: the type of cancer, its size and location in the body and the kind of cells it contains (commonly called the stage), as well as the patient's overall state of health, are all important parameters in the choice of the best treatment strategy. Most of the time, the surgical removal of tumors, radiotherapy and chemotherapy are used simultaneously or sequentially. For example, surgical removal of a tumor is a fairly common procedure, followed

## The six hallmarks of cancer

1. Unregulated growth allowing cancer cells to reproduce even in the absence of biochemical signals.
2. Refusal to obey antigrowth commands issued by cells nearby that perceive the danger to the tissue.
3. Resistance to suicide by apoptosis, thus evading the control of the cell-protection mechanisms.
4. Ability to cause new blood vessels to form through angiogenesis, so that oxygen and nutrients essential to growth can be supplied.
5. Acquisition of all of these characteristics so as to make cancer cells immortal and thus able to replicate themselves indefinitely.
6. Ability to invade and colonize the organism's tissues, first locally and then by spreading as metastases.

by radiotherapy or chemotherapy treatment to eliminate residual cancer cells.

Despite the considerable progress made as a result of these therapeutic approaches, cancer remains a very difficult disease to treat. These difficulties can be attributed to three major limits of current therapies.

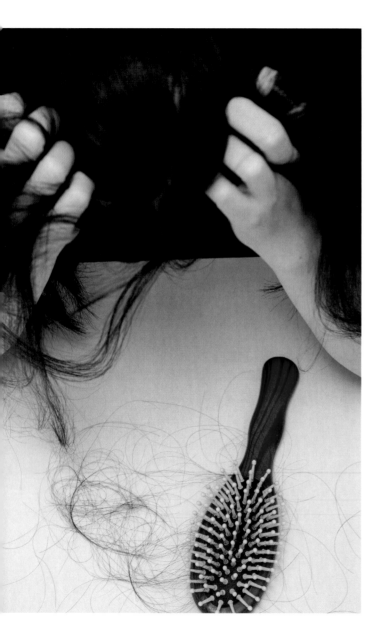

*Side effects.* One of the main problems with chemotherapy drugs is their toxicity for many healthy cells in the body, which causes multiple side effects. These include a decrease in immune cells and platelets, anemia, digestive disorders (nausea, attacks on the digestive mucosa) and hair loss (alopecia), not to mention various cardiac, renal and other complications. As a result, the length of treatment is often limited by these side effects, making it sometimes impossible to eliminate the cancer cells completely. What's more, some of the chemotherapy drugs used in treating certain tumors cause DNA mutations; they are thus by definition carcinogenic and can increase the risk of cancer in the short or long term.

*Resistance.* While, generally speaking, all cancers are greatly reduced or even eradicated by chemotherapy or radiotherapy (we say in these cases that the tumors "respond" to treatment), tumors nonetheless often recur after a period of time. These recurrences are usually a bad sign, for these new tumors have often become resistant to a broad range of treatments. In the case of chemotherapy, for example, a mechanism often used by tumor cells to adapt to the poison is the production of specific proteins that "pump" the drugs out of the cell and thus prevent them from doing any damage. Another mechanism consists of disposing of genes that would compel them to commit suicide when the drug enters the cell. In short, even when a chemotherapy treatment succeeds in killing 99.9 percent of the cancer cells, all it takes is for a single one to have successfully acquired a new trait giving it resistance to the drug for the tumor to recur, this time composed of clones of that tumor cell, even more dangerous than the cells in the earlier tumor. As we have said, we should not perhaps be too surprised at the ability of cancer cells to adapt; this adaptation mechanism is at the heart of life on Earth. Even less evolved cells are often able to find ways to resist obstacles in their path, as witnessed in the resurgence of a number of diseases associated with bacteria resistant to several classes of antibiotics.

*Tumor heterogeneity.* There are major differences in tumor composition, both among different individuals and within a single cancer. Analysis of the various anatomical regions of a lung cancer, for example, reveals the presence of several different genetic defects that have all evolved in their own way. In other words, a cancerous mass is not just one cancer, but rather a combination of several cancers, each containing several million completely degenerated cells (Figure 12). Similarly, what we call "breast cancer" is really a generic term referring to a family of at least 10 distinct diseases, each with its own molecular imprint and specific characteristics. Cancer's considerable heterogeneity thus

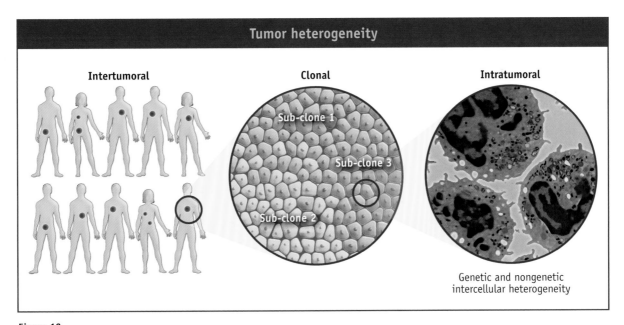

**Tumor heterogeneity**

Intertumoral

Clonal

Sub-clone 1

Sub-clone 3

Sub-clone 2

Intratumoral

Genetic and nongenetic intercellular heterogeneity

**Figure 12**

means that even if a given treatment manages to neutralize an oncogene that promotes cancer growth, the tumor is likely to contain subpopulations of cells that use other means to grow and will be resistant to this treatment. As a result, even new anticancer therapies that specifically target certain genetic abnormalities in tumors are often powerless to cure a majority of patients, despite the often exorbitant costs associated with these drugs.

All of these factors illustrate what an incredibly complex disease mature cancer is, and how extremely difficult it is to treat it successfully. It is important to realize, however, that the appearance of a tumor is in no way an instant development, but rather the result of a long process occurring over many years, in which the cell, "awakened" by the appearance of an error in its genetic material, transforms itself completely to overcome the many obstacles encountered in the course of its development. The most important aspect of this long process is that, for many years, even decades, cancer cells remain extremely vulnerable and only a few of them successfully reach the malignant stage. This vulnerability means it is possible to interfere at several points in the tumor's development and thus prevent cancer from appearing. We will emphasize this point throughout this book, as this notion is key to reducing deaths from cancer: the tumor must be attacked while it is vulnerable if we really want to reduce the number of cases of cancer in our societies. By rediscovering, so to speak, its ancestors' original instincts, designed to ensure its autonomous survival, the tumor cell acquires fearsome power. And this is what makes cancer so hard to fight: trying to destroy these primitive cells is like trying to eliminate the adaptive force that created us. We are fighting the forces at the very origins of life.

**In summary:**

- Cancer is a disease caused by the disruption of cellular functions, in which the cell gradually acquires characteristics allowing it to grow and invade the organism's tissues.

- The acquisition of these cancerous properties occurs over a long period of time, during a latency period that offers a golden opportunity to intervene to prevent tumors from reaching a mature stage.

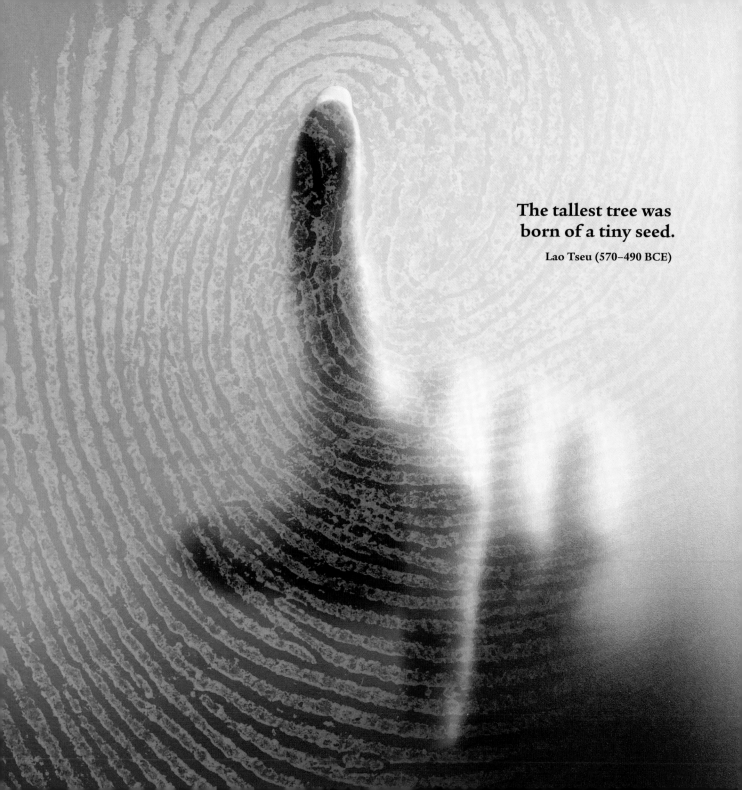

The tallest tree was
born of a tiny seed.

Lao Tseu (570–490 BCE)

# Chapter 3

# Cancer Is an Environmental Issue... for Cells

In the armor of tumor cells, is there a chink that could enhance our chances of defeating them? The answer is yes. A cancer cell, despite its power, adaptability and genetic instability, cannot by itself succeed in invading the tissues in which it lives; it must rely on an environment favorable to this growth, a welcoming milieu that will provide it with the elements essential to its progression and support the constant quest for mutations needed to achieve its conquering aims. Preventing the creation of this kind of procarcinogenic environment is absolutely essential to effectively stop cancer from developing.

## A seed in soil

The development of cancer can in a way be compared to that of a seed in soil; the seed appears vulnerable at first glance, but when conditions are favorable it has the incredible ability to take advantage of all of the soil's resources to grow to maturity (Figure 13). In the case of a plant, we know that the seed must be able to rely on an adequate supply of sun and water, two factors indispensable for the assimilation of the nutrients in the soil. The same is true for cancer: precancerous cells, whether they are hereditary in origin or acquired during our lifetime, are incapable on their own of taking advantage of the resources in their environment. In fact, this environment (called the stroma) is composed of a very large number of noncancerous cells, in particular the cells in the conjunctive tissue, an environment that is not very receptive to precancerous cells and even has an anticancer effect that limits their development. The evolution of these precancerous cells thus depends totally on additional factors that will "activate" the stroma and force it to modify its status quo so the cells can obtain the elements they need to progress.

Two types of procarcinogenic factors in cells' immediate environment are especially important for cancer development. The first, which can in some respects be compared to water, aims to root the seed more solidly in the soil, so that it can become established and gain access to a constant supply of nutrients. To do this, cancer cells produce chemical signals, notably VEGF, to attract cells from a blood vessel located nearby. By attaching itself to a receptor on the surface of the vessel's cells, VEGF enables these cells to migrate toward the tumor by dissolving the surrounding tissue and creating enough new cells to produce a new blood vessel. This process, called *tumoral angiogenesis* (from the Greek *angio,* vessel, and *genesis*, creation), thus contributes to the tumor's progression by providing it with a new network of blood vessels to meet its energy needs and continue to invade surrounding tissues (Figure 14).

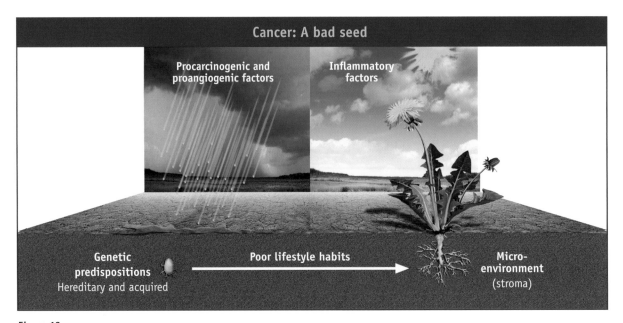

Figure 13

The growth stimulated by procarcinogenic and proangiogenic factors would be much slower, however, if the immature tumor could not count on another kind of procarcinogenic factor, which, just like sunshine in the case of a plant, speeds up the process by supplying it with an important source of powerful stimulators: the inflammatory cells in our immune system. In other words, like water and sunshine for plants, these procarcinogenic and inflammatory factors act together to enable precancerous cells to draw on the elements needed for their progression in their immediate environment.

## Cancer, an inflammatory disease

Inflammation caused by our immune system is essential to our body's integrity; without it, we would be completely at the mercy of the many pathogenic agents in our environment (see box, p. 44). But when it becomes too intense or occurs over too long a period, inflammation can cause several medical conditions to develop and even promote the progression of diseases like cancer. A close relationship between inflammation and cancer was already recognized by the first pathologists who took an interest in cancer. In fact, the presence of a large number of

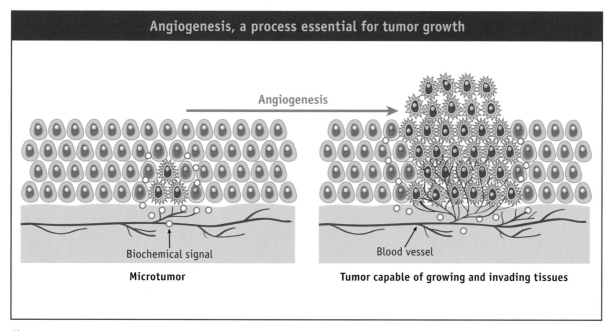

**Angiogenesis, a process essential for tumor growth**

Angiogenesis

Biochemical signal

Blood vessel

**Microtumor**

**Tumor capable of growing and invading tissues**

**Figure 14**

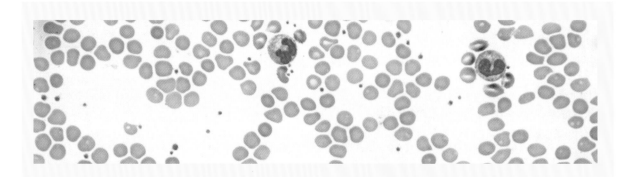

## Inflammation, an ally that can also become an enemy...

The immune system consists of everything that defends us from attacks, whether pathogenic (bacteria, viruses), chemical or traumatic in origin. This system is an armed force composed of elite soldiers divided into groups specializing in very specific neutralization or attack activities. The "inflammatory squad," the division responsible for quickly neutralizing intruders, is the first responder. The cells of this squad, especially the white blood cells known as macrophages, are called "inflammatory" because they release highly reactive molecules designed to eliminate any pathogenic agents that might try to invade our body; this causes irritation (easily recognizable as rashes, swellings or itching). This inflammatory reaction also helps to begin repairing damaged tissues, owing to the many growth factors secreted by the inflammatory cells that in turn speed up the arrival of healthy cells and encourage the formation of new blood vessels. Normally, this reaction should not last long, since the continued presence of inflammatory molecules becomes extremely irritating for the affected tissues. When they linger, a state of chronic inflammation takes hold, which can cause intense pain in the inflamed area. As we will see, chronic inflammation can also be the result of a number of lifestyle factors (smoking, obesity, too many calories, omega-3 fatty acid deficiency). Although this kind of chronic inflammation does not necessarily cause obvious symptoms, it nonetheless creates a favorable environment for the growth of cells in the inflamed area; this is especially dangerous if the tissue contains microtumors made up of precancerous cells. These can then use the growth factors secreted by the inflammatory cells, as well as the new blood vessel network created near the inflammation, to become a mature tumor.

macrophages and other immune cells in tumors is a fundamental characteristic of many cancers (we should stress that, in general, the greater the number of these cells, the more advanced and dangerous the tumor has become).

The importance of inflammation in the development of cancer is also clearly illustrated by the close relationship between various diseases caused by chronic inflammation and the dramatic increase in cancer risk associated with these inflammatory diseases. In fact, it has long been known that chronic inflammation, whether caused by repeated exposure to toxic products (cigarette smoke, asbestos fibers), by certain bacteria or viruses (*Helicobacter pylori*, the hepatitis virus) or by a long-term metabolic imbalance, considerably increases the risk of developing cancer in the organs affected by these inflammatory attacks (Figure 15). For example, inflammation caused by the continued presence of *H. pylori* in the stomach increases the risk of cancer in this organ by three to six times, while ulcerative colitis, a chronic inflammatory disease of the large intestine, increases the risk of colon cancer by nearly 10 times. These relationships are far from being isolated cases: overall, it is estimated that chronic inflammatory diseases are directly linked to one in every six cancers worldwide.

| Inflammatory diseases that predispose to cancer | |
|---|---|
| Inflammatory intestinal disease | **Colorectal cancer** |
| Gastritis caused by *H. pylori* | **Stomach cancer** |
| Pelvic inflammatory disease | **Ovarian cancer** |
| Schistosomiasis | **Bladder cancer** |
| *H. pylori* | **MALT lymphoma** |
| Hepatitis viruses B and C | **Liver cancer** |
| HHV-8 | **Kaposi sarcoma** |
| Silicosis | **Bronchial cancer** |
| Asbestosis | **Mesothelioma** |
| Barrett's metaplasia | **Esophageal cancer** |
| Thyroiditis | **Papillary thyroid cancer** |
| Prostatitis | **Prostate cancer** |

Figure 15

## Inflammation lights the spark!

The mechanisms by which precancerous cells use inflammation to progress to a mature stage are complex and attest to cancer's extraordinary ability to make use of all the elements in its immediate environment to achieve its goals.

For example, cancer cells secrete messages aimed at inflammatory cells located nearby, forcing them to release a large number of growth factors and enzymes. These allow the cancer cells to make their way through the tissue structure, along with certain molecules essential for the formation of the network of blood vessels required for cancer progression (Figure 16). All of these factors normally serve to speed up healing and re-establish the damaged tissues' equilibrium, but for a precancerous tumor trying to improve its chances of growth, these tools are a godsend!

These factors also help cancer cells survive by activating a key protein with the delightful name "nuclear factor-κB" (NF-κB), which also plays a crucial role in the growth of these cells by increasing the production of cyclooxygenase-2 (COX-2), a very important enzyme involved in the production of inflammatory molecules. The excess COX-2 leads to an increase in macrophages and immune cells at the inflammation site. The result is the creation of a vicious circle in which growth factors produced by the macrophages are used by the cancer cells to survive and progress; at the same time, the survival of the cancer cells causes large amounts of inflammatory molecules to be produced, thus creating a favorable climate for recruiting other macrophages. This is why inflammation is a key element in cancer progression: by creating an environment rich

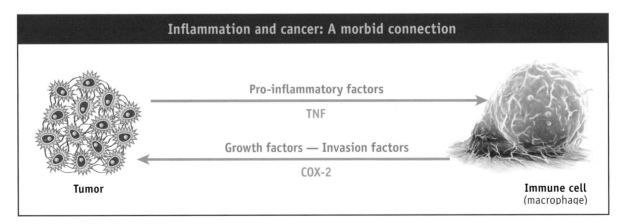

**Inflammation and cancer: A morbid connection**

Pro-inflammatory factors

TNF

Growth factors — Invasion factors

COX-2

**Tumor**

**Immune cell**
(macrophage)

**Figure 16**

in growth factors, the continued presence of inflammatory cells provides precancerous cells with ideal conditions so they can speed up their attempts to mutate and acquire new properties essential for continuing their progression.

## Obesity: Inflammation carries weight

The chronic inflammation so essential for cancer development is not always caused by attacks from outside; lifestyle can also play a major role. The most important contributor to the creation of this kind of inflammatory environment is without a doubt too much body fat: when they are overloaded with fat, the cells making up the fatty tissue (the adipocytes) behave like magnets and attract inflammatory cells from the immune system, as well as some classes of lymphocytes; this causes low-level chronic inflammation that is invisible and undetectable, but that nonetheless disrupts the body's overall equilibrium (Figure 17).

The contribution of inflammation caused by excess weight to cancer development is clearly illustrated by the significant increase in the incidence of the disease and the mortality associated with it in overweight people, an especially pronounced impact for cancers of the uterus, esophagus, kidney, colon and breast (Figure 18). On the whole, it is estimated that

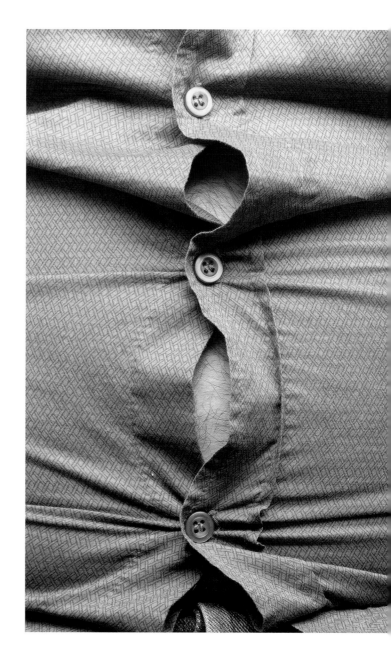

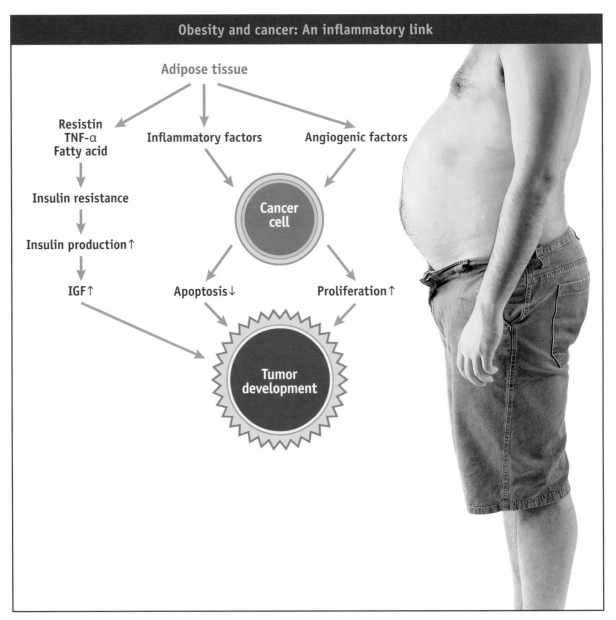

**Obesity and cancer: An inflammatory link**

Adipose tissue

Resistin
TNF-α
Fatty acid

Inflammatory factors

Angiogenic factors

Insulin resistance

Insulin production↑

IGF↑

Cancer cell

Apoptosis↓

Proliferation↑

Tumor development

**Figure 17**

Adapted from Calle and Kaaks, 2004.

excess weight and obesity are responsible for cancers in half a million people worldwide. Women are especially vulnerable, since excess weight is associated with a very large increase in cancers of the endometrium, colon and breast (postmenopause). In men, colon and kidney cancers alone represent two-thirds of cancers related to being overweight.

These statistics are alarming, as excess weight and obesity have more or less become the norm in most industrialized countries. In Canada, two out of every three people are overweight and, according to criteria established by the World Health Organization, approximately one billion people in the world are carrying too much weight (body mass index

higher than 25), with 312 million of them, of whom roughly 30 million are children, being obese (body mass index higher than 30). This is an unprecedented public health crisis that risks worsening in the coming years, since carrying excess weight affects a growing proportion of children, who are at much greater risk of retaining this extra weight in adulthood.

Strangely, instead of reacting and doing everything possible to contain this crisis, our society seems resigned to this explosion of excess weight and obesity, somewhat as if it were a new "trend" we have to come to terms with to avoid stigmatizing overweight people. This fatalistic view is very dangerous, however, because excess weight and obesity are not

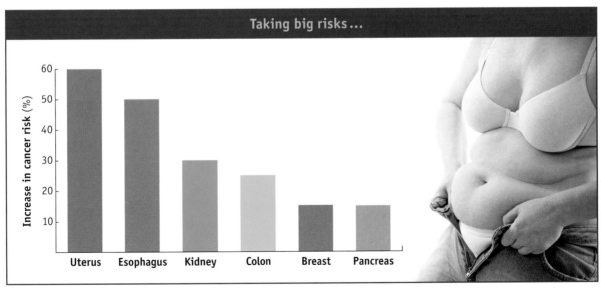

Taking big risks…

**Figure 18**

Adapted from M.J. Khandekar et al., 2011.

aesthetic problems, but rather completely abnormal physiological states, which cause major disruption to the body's equilibrium and impose huge constraints on the entire human body.

The chronic inflammation associated with excess body fat means therefore that excess weight must be considered a carcinogenic agent just like tobacco, alcohol and UV rays. Carrying too much fat anywhere, especially in the abdomen, should be viewed as a warning signal, a visible manifestation of significant changes in the equilibrium of our vital functions that increase our risk for several diseases, including cancer.

## Shutting the door on cancer

All of these observations indicate that to prevent cancer the cellular environment of precancerous cells absolutely has to be modified, to keep it from nurturing elements likely to create a favorable climate for tumor growth.

It is important to understand that this principle applies to all precancerous cells, whether they stem from heredity, are formed by exposure to a carcinogenic substance or are simply the result of bad luck (Figure 19). For example, a person born with a defective gene will have precancerous cells very early in his or her life (the "seed"), but these immature tumors will generally not be able to grow unless they can rely on the presence of "soil" that encourages this growth. Thus, women carrying a mutation of the BRCA gene are at higher risk of developing breast and ovarian cancer, but this risk is considerably increased by lifestyle factors that create favorable conditions for tumor progression, in particular a poor diet and excess body weight. The same goes for the increase in cancer risk that accompanies aging:

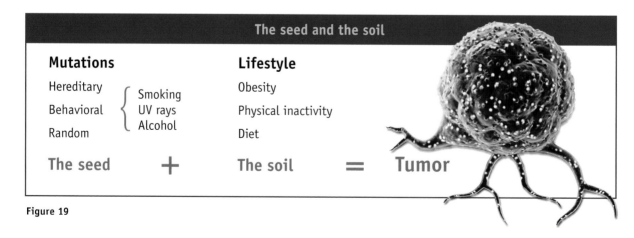

**The seed and the soil**

**Mutations**

Hereditary

Behavioral { Smoking, UV rays, Alcohol

Random

**Lifestyle**

Obesity

Physical inactivity

Diet

**The seed** + **The soil** = **Tumor**

**Figure 19**

the accumulation of spontaneous genetic errors during a lifetime significantly increases the number of immature tumors in the organs, but their development into mature cancers can be greatly encouraged by lifestyle. Kidney and esophageal cancers, for example, have increased more than sixfold in the last 40 years, regardless of the age of those affected, a consequence once again of bad diet and weight gain. In short, even when there is a serious genetic predisposition or an accumulation of spontaneous genetic errors as we age, lifestyle remains the factor that wields the greatest influence over our risk of getting the disease.

To keep cancer from getting a foothold, chronic inflammation must first be kept as low as possible. In recent years, several studies have shown that those who habitually took anti-inflammatory drugs that specifically inhibited COX-2 activity had a lower risk of getting some types of cancer, especially colon cancer. However, these drugs have significant side effects for the cardiovascular system (which even led to Vioxx being taken off the market), which limits their preventive use. Nonetheless, the protective effect of these anti-inflammatory molecules indicates that reducing inflammation represents a very promising approach in cancer prevention.

In addition to excess weight and obesity, eating too many processed foods, overloaded with sugars and harmful fats, and not enough plant-based products, especially fruits and vegetables, are factors likely to create inflammatory conditions favorable to cancer development.

Preventing the formation of new blood vessels through angiogenesis is another aspect that must be considered. It is now well established that in the absence of new blood vessels, tumors cannot grow larger than 1 mm$^3$, too small to cause irreparable damage to the surrounding tissues. Preventing the neovascularization of tumors that have not yet begun to grow completely independently — immature tumors in a latent state in the organism — might therefore be a highly effective strategy for preventing the development of cancer. Furthermore, since the vast majority of tumors depend on an adequate blood supply, inhibiting the formation of these new vessels can prevent the development of some cancers. Even liquid tumors, like leukemias, require bone marrow vascularization and are therefore likely to be targeted by these treatments.

To sum up, cancer growth must be viewed not as an isolated event, but as a process whose success depends directly on favorable conditions supplied by the host. Cancer's heavy reliance on its environment is, however, a weakness, a chink in its armor that can be exploited. Cancer creates nothing — it is a by nature a parasite that remains in a fragile state

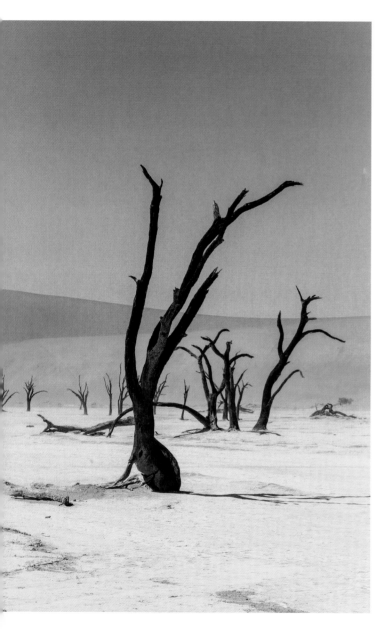

as long as it finds itself in. When conditions are in its favor, as we have seen, it deploys its reserves of ingenuity to make use of its immediate environment for its own benefit, constantly searching for new mutations that will allow it to grow. On the other hand, in the absence of favorable conditions, cancer is weakened and cannot express its full potential. It is condemned to remain inconspicuous, anonymous and powerless.

Preventing cancer by reducing inflammation and inhibiting angiogenesis is not a dream — it already happens. Some of the foods we eat, especially plants, are prime sources of anti-inflammatory and antiangiogenic compounds which, taken daily, create a climate hostile to cancer progression. Because of this preventive approach, cancer is no longer a fatal disease. Instead, it is a chronic disease whose control requires constant treatment.

**In summary:**

- Chronic inflammation participates actively in cancer growth by encouraging the survival and growth of precancerous cells, as well as by allowing them to acquire a network of blood vessels to supply their energy needs.

- Excess weight and obesity encourage the establishment of this pro-inflammatory environment and thus increase the risk of developing several types of cancer.

- Regularly eating plant-based foods and maintaining a normal body weight play a crucial role in reducing inflammation and angiogenesis, both indispensable to cancer prevention.

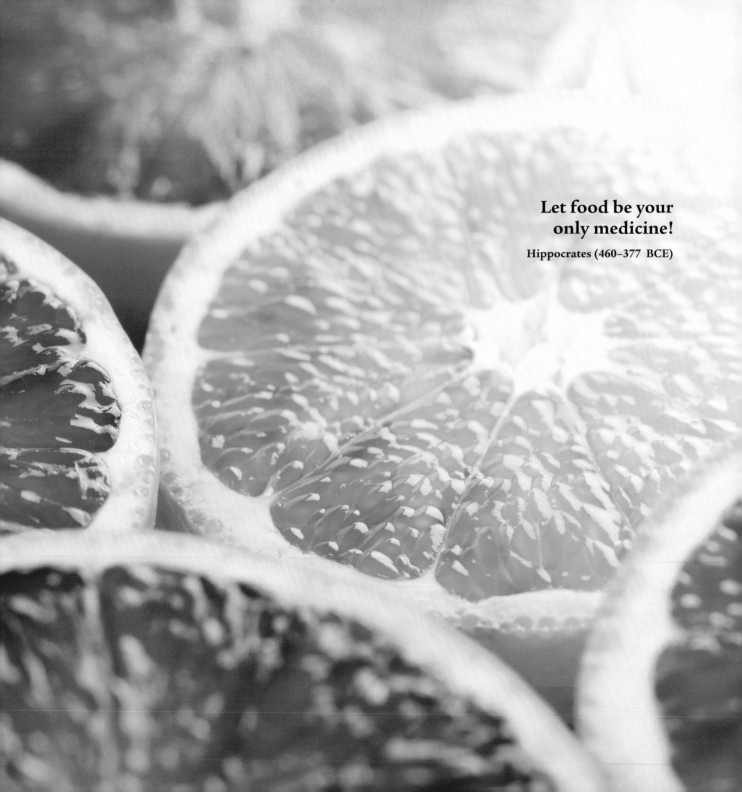

Let food be your
only medicine!

Hippocrates (460–377 BCE)

# Chapter 4

# Preventing Cancer Through Diet

The high proportion of cancers attributable to the nature of the Western diet is, as we have seen, a sign of a deterioration in food habits in a society that has lost contact with the very idea of diet and that sees the act of eating only as an activity designed to supply energy to the body, without regard for its impact on health. This kind of mindless diet, based purely and simply on satisfying the need to eat, is most certainly harmful to health. In an era when we often have a tendency to consider progress to be a synonym for benefit, it must be said that this relationship does not hold true in the case of diet, and that industrialization is in the process of destroying the very basis of our dietary culture.

Everything we know today about the nutritional or toxic properties of a plant, or about using certain foods for therapeutic purposes, is the result of human beings' long quest during the course of their evolution to determine the value and quality of foods located in their immediate environment. What we call a "fruit" or "vegetable" is precisely the result of a selection process that took place over a period of 15 million years, during which humanoids adapted to changes in their environment, constantly on the lookout for new food sources, new vegetable species that could give them a better chance of survival. Diet as we now know it is thus a very recent concept: if we transposed the history of 15 million years of the diet of human beings and their ancestors to a 365-day calendar, agriculture, which is a mere 8,000 years old, would only have been invented on December 31 around 7 p.m., while the industrialization of food, even more recent, would only appear three minutes before the New Year (Figure 20). Emphasizing the crucial importance of plants for maintaining good health is therefore not at all original or revolutionary: in practice, these foods have been a part of our diet for 15 million years! Viewed from this angle, it is not surprising that a deficiency of plants, typical of the current diet in Western countries, can have such harmful effects on health.

## Plants à la carte

The food selection process can be visualized in three main stages (Figure 21). During the first stage, which could be called "the study of toxicity," the first humans were forced to make many attempts to find out if the plants available to them were edible. A dangerous enterprise, of course, which no doubt led to serious poisonings, and even deaths, in the case of plants that were especially harmful because of their poison content. Obviously, in many cases, observing other animals could prove useful and prevent accidents (it is highly likely

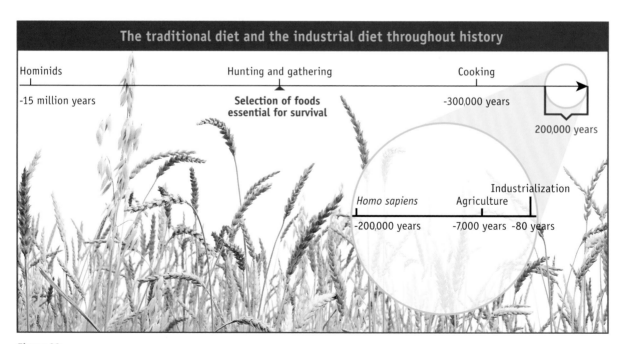

**Figure 20**

that the idea of eating oysters would never have occurred to humans if they had not seen sea otters doing so), but a great deal of trial and error was no doubt necessary to determine which plants did not cause physical disorders and could be considered nontoxic and edible. This knowledge was obviously transmitted to the immediate family as well as to other members of the community — otherwise, all these efforts would have quite useless.

During the second stage of the selection process, which could be called "the evaluation stage," nontoxic plants chosen initially were included in the diet, but continued to be "under observation," for, despite being nontoxic, many did not really have any benefits for the organism, either because they contained toxins or drugs that could endanger survival in the long-term, or because they did not provide anything nutritious or positive for health. Eating grass may not be toxic, but it is not a useful food source for humans.

Finally, the third stage, called "the selection stage," was where foods that offer real benefit to the organism were chosen, either because of their nutrient supply, or because of the observation of the additional health benefits provided by eating them. After all, human beings do not just want to eat to live; they want their life to be as pleasant and long as possible. This quest for longevity led them to seek benefits in their diet over and above just

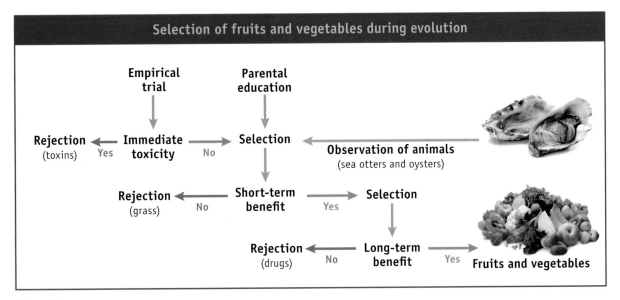

Figure 21

nutrient supply, for the simple reason that it was the only resource they had that was likely to have an influence on their health and prolong their lives. We should not therefore be surprised that the history of medicine is inseparable from that of diet, since diet was, for a long time, human beings' only medicine.

The great ancient civilizations — Egyptian, Indian, Chinese and Greek — all recorded in very detailed texts their observations on the positive effects of plants and foods on health, as well as their curative properties. The importance of diet as a way to maintain health was actually the basis of all medical approaches until the beginning of the 20th century. Much more than a simple question of survival, acquiring this knowledge of what is good, bad or neutral for health is a cultural heritage of inestimable value illustrating the fundamental relationship uniting humans, nature and food.

If we tried to imitate the ancients by writing a book today on foods that are good for health, not many foods currently popular in the West would deserve to be included. It is this total break with the past that explains why, in an era when medicine has never been more powerful, we are witnessing the emergence of diseases that were very rare barely a century ago, like colon cancer. Lessons can be learned, however, from knowledge dating back thousands of years based on the observation of nature and plants. Making use of this knowledge, in combination with modern medicine, cannot help but have extraordinary repercussions for our health, especially in terms of cancer prevention.

Recent research has demonstrated that some of the foods selected by humans in the course of their evolution contain countless molecules with anticancer potential that can genuinely help reduce the incidence of cancer. Western societies' current lack of interest in the nature of their diet is therefore not just a simple break with dietary culture, but, even worse, the rejection of an outstanding source of very potent anticancer molecules.

## Plants, an abundant source of anticancer agents

The recognition of the therapeutic potential of many plants dates back to very ancient times: even our distant ancestors the chimpanzees are capable of identifying plant species with medicinal properties able to effectively fight some of their diseases (see box, p. 59)!

## What is a food?

A food is a product eaten regularly by a group that has recognized its harmlessness and long-term benefits for health.

Research carried out in recent years has highlighted the fact that a large number of plants and foodstuffs that are part of the daily diet of many cultures are exceptional sources of molecules with the ability to interfere with some of the processes at work in cancer development, in a way similar to the mode of action of many drugs used today.

Drugs, whether for cancer or other diseases, are always molecules able to interrupt an absolutely essential stage in the development of a disease, a kind of switch that, once turned off, prevents the disease from developing. Since, in the vast majority of cases, disorders in the functioning of a class of specialized proteins, or enzymes, are responsible for diseases like cancer, it goes without saying that most drugs aim to block the functioning of these enzymes to re-establish a kind of equilibrium and prevent the disease from progressing. For example, if an enzyme has to interact with a given substance for a disease to progress, the drug will often try to imitate the structure of this substance so as to block its access to the enzyme and thus limit the enzyme's functioning (Figure 22). The molecules that manage to block the enzyme's activity by acting as a decoy may not only

## Pharmacist Chimpanzees

Not only are herbivorous animals able to identify toxic plants and avoid eating them, but some of them, in particular chimpanzees, are able to choose certain plant families to treat their infections. For example, chimpanzees with intestinal upsets eat the young shoots of a small tree not usually consumed by these monkeys because of its strong bitterness. A very wise choice, as a biological analysis of this plant has uncovered several antiparasitic compounds that had never before been isolated! Other studies have shown that, following an injury, chimpanzees eat the stems of a thorny plant (*Acanthus pubescens*), as well as the fruit and leaves of some species of *Ficus*. These choices would certainly have been approved by the region's physician-healers, since these plants are all used in local medicine to treat injuries and ulcers! The use of plants for curative purposes thus goes back to the dawn of humanity, which shows just how much our close relationship with the plant world around us shaped the evolution of our species.

be synthetic; they may also occur naturally in foods that are part of our daily diet. For example, a molecule found in large quantity in soy, genistein (see Chapter 8), is extremely similar to estradiol, an estrogenic female sex hormone — hence its name "phytoestrogen" (Figure 23).

Because of this resemblance, genistein acts as a decoy for the protein, which normally recognizes estradiol, and can fill the place usually taken by this hormone, thus reducing the impact of estradiol's biological effects, notably the growth of tissues sensitive to this hormone, like breast tissues. Genistein's mode of action even compares with that of tamoxifen, a drug prescribed for many years for breast cancer. This example shows the extent to which some foods contain molecules with structures and mechanisms analogous to those of several synthetic drugs, and how useful they can be in preventing diseases like cancer.

The main difference between the molecules in foods and synthetic molecules is not so much related to their effectiveness as to their source (plant or synthetic), as well as to the way they have been selected by humans. As we have seen, in the case of foods, this process required a very long selection process, whereas for synthetic molecules the time scale is much shorter, which makes evaluating the possible side effects difficult.

The selection of foods by humans that we described earlier is somewhat comparable to the evaluation of the toxicity of synthetic molecules, except that the evaluation of foods took place over several million years, a length of time that

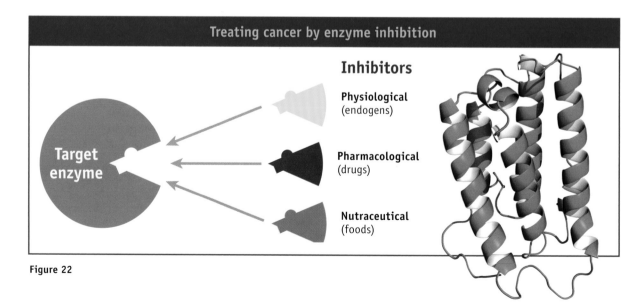

**Treating cancer by enzyme inhibition**

**Inhibitors**

**Physiological** (endogens)

**Pharmacological** (drugs)

**Nutraceutical** (foods)

Target enzyme

Figure 22

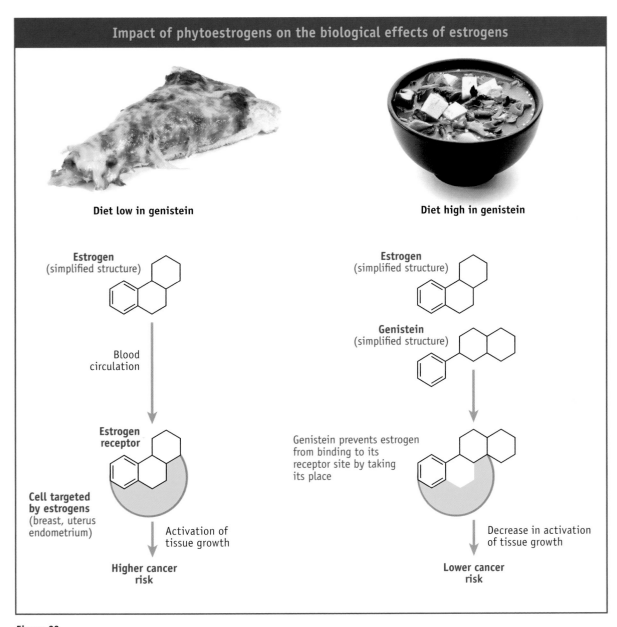

**Figure 23**

# A plant pharmacy

The plant world contains a bank of compounds with healthful properties, with many of them being especially active against cancer cells. Some of these complex anticancer plant molecules are very effective and can be used just as they are (taxol, vincristine, vinblastine) to treat advanced cancer, or act as a starting point for producing event more powerful derivatives (etoposide, irinotecan, docetaxel). The therapeutic use of plant-sourced anticancer molecules is far from insignificant, given that over 60 percent of chemotherapy drugs still in clinical use that make it possible to save many lives come in one way or another from plant sources!

made it possible to exclude all forms of toxicity potentially associated with a food; anticancer molecules in this food do not therefore have undesirable side effects. Conversely, in spite of all precautions, a synthetic molecule is completely foreign to the organism, with the inherent risk of causing undesirable side effects, as is almost always the case. So, although there are many analogies between the modes of action of nutritional and synthetic molecules, the basic difference between the two approaches is the absence of toxicity associated with the consumption of anticancer molecules naturally found in fruits and vegetables (Figure 24). In fact, molecules originating in food have the ability to interact with most of the targets that synthetic drugs developed by industry aim at, illustrating yet again the extent to which

## Pharmacological and nutritional anticancer agents

| Pharmacological molecules | Nutritional molecules | |
|---|---|---|
| • Known chemical structures | • Known chemical structures | 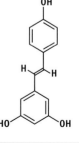 |
| • Well-established cellular and molecular targets | • Well-established cellular and molecular targets | |
| • Synthetic | • Natural | |
| • Selected in a laboratory | • Selected during evolution | |
| • Sometimes very pronounced side effects | • No side effects | |
| • Synergy or antagonism seldom observed and randomly caused | • Synergy or antagonism selected during evolution | |

Figure 24

foods can have positive impacts on health (Figure 25).

The anticancer properties associated with compounds in foods of plant origin are not at all abstract or theoretical; on the contrary, molecules able to interfere with cancer development are widely found in plants, so much so that most chemotherapy drugs currently used come from plant sources (see box). In the same vein, a number of compounds of nutritional origin that have an inhibiting activity on specific processes associated with cancer development are currently used as models for the pharmaceutical industry, with the aim of producing analogue molecules for use in treating cancer.

Encouraging the increased consumption of foods rich in anticancer molecules to prevent cancer comes down to drawing on new possibilities for therapeutic intervention, from a bank of compounds developed by nature over 3.8 billion years through a process of trial and error similar to that used by the pharmaceutical industry to discover new drugs to successfully treat various diseases.

## Preventive chemotherapy

The use of molecules occurring in our daily diet is even more important because we are constantly running the risk of developing

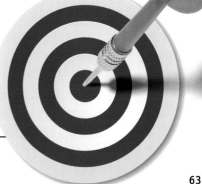

**Pharmacological targets of phytochemical compounds**

- Tumoral invasion and metastases inhibition
- Growth factor receptor inhibition
- Inflammatory enzyme (COX-2) inhibition
- Transcription factor inhibition
- Chemotherapy drug resistance inhibition
- Platelet aggregation inhibition
- Antiestrogens
- Antibacterial action
- Immune system modulation
- Cellular signal cascade inhibition
- Toxicity to cancer cells
- Cancer cell cytoskeleton perturbation
- Toxin metabolic action inhibition via Phase I (cytochrome P450)
- Toxin detoxification activation via Phase II

**Figure 25**

tumors, and, by using the anticancer molecules in food, these tumors can be maintained in a latent state (see box). Another factor that makes preventive therapy for cancer through food important is that people's genes are very different. All human beings possess roughly the same genes (otherwise we would not belong to the same species), but there are nonetheless significant variations that dictate each individual's distinct characteristics. These variations are not only responsible for the noticeable physical differences among people, but also affect other genes, which, if they are inactivated, can make some people less able to defend themselves from attacks, like those caused by carcinogenic substances.

Even though a limited proportion of cancers are transmissible by heredity, several genetic factors do make some people much more likely to develop cancer, following their exposure to carcinogenic agents, for example, and their need to protect themselves by consuming anticancer molecules is that much greater. This concept was brilliantly illustrated by the results of a study done in Shanghai, in which individuals lacking two enzymes important for eliminating toxic aggressors ran three times the risk of getting lung cancer if their diet did not contain cruciferous vegetables. On the other hand, other people with the same mutations, but who ate large amounts of these vegetables, had a lower risk of cancer in comparison with the general population. These observations show the extent to which diet enables us to mitigate the impact of genetic disorders that increase people's susceptibility to developing cancers.

It bears repeating: fighting cancer development through diet means using the anticancer molecules in certain foods as weapons to create an environment hostile to these tumors, so as to bombard tumor sites on a daily basis and prevent tumor growth — just like chemotherapy.

The human body must be viewed as a battlefield where there is an

| We all have tumors | | |
| --- | --- | --- |
| Organs | Tumors found during autopsy (%) | Tumors diagnosed clinically (%) |
| **Breast** (women 40–50) | 33 | 1 |
| **Prostate** (men 40–50) | 40 | 2 |
| **Thyroid** | 98 | 0.1 |

Figure 26

# Cancer: A chronic disease

It is important to realize that tumor formation is a random event that is relatively frequent in an individual's lifetime. Pathology studies have shown that a very large proportion of people who have died from causes other than cancer had microtumors that had not been clinically detected in their tissues. In one of these studies, 98 percent of people had small tumors in the thyroid, 40 percent in the prostate and 33 percent in the breast, whereas tumors in these organs are only normally detected in a small percentage of the population (Figure 26). Similarly, even though Asian men have in general a prostate cancer rate several times lower than that of Western men, the analysis of biopsies carried out on Asian and Western populations shows that the number of cells in the prostate in the process of acquiring cancerous properties (precancerous cells) is exactly the same in both populations, indicating that lifestyle habits, including diet, are determining factors in whether or not these microtumors reach a clinical stage.

Our natural defenses ensure that tumors that form spontaneously inside us usually remain microscopic, posing no danger to health. A continuous intake of anti-inflammatory and antiangiogenetic molecules from the diet assists the body's natural defenses and helps maintain tumors in a harmless state. Thus, even though

we constantly run the risk of developing cancer, the use of anticancer molecules in food as a therapeutic weapon is an approach essential for keeping these tumors in a latent state and preventing them from progressing to the advanced cancer stage. Cancer must therefore be viewed as a chronic disease that can be controlled in daily life with the help of foods high in anticancer compounds.

Regular consumption of fruits and vegetables is like preventive chemotherapy; it keeps microtumors from reaching a stage with pathological consequences and it is nontoxic for the physiology of normal tissues. Diet's preventive role is not restricted to preventing cancer's appearance (primary prevention); it also makes it possible to thwart the growth of residual cancer cells that might have avoided chemotherapy treatment and could again develop into tumors (recurrence), once again threatening the life of a person with the disease.

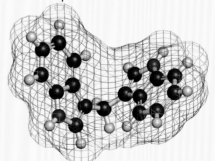

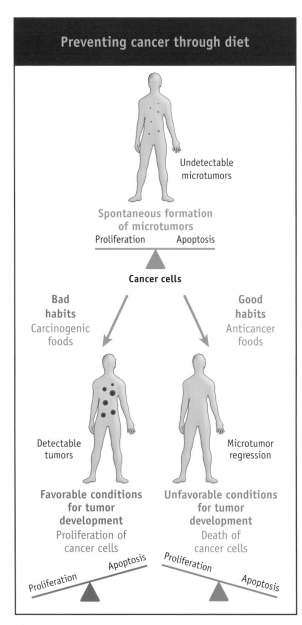

**Preventing cancer through diet**

Undetectable microtumors

Spontaneous formation of microtumors

Proliferation    Apoptosis

**Cancer cells**

**Bad habits**
Carcinogenic foods

**Good habits**
Anticancer foods

Detectable tumors

Microtumor regression

**Favorable conditions for tumor development**
Proliferation of cancer cells

**Unfavorable conditions for tumor development**
Death of cancer cells

Proliferation    Apoptosis

Proliferation    Apoptosis

**Figure 27**

ongoing fight between mutant cells trying to develop into autonomous entities and to turn into cancer, and our defense mechanisms trying to preserve the body's integrity. To go back to the image of the switch, a diet consisting mainly of bad foods, or lacking in protective foods like fruits and vegetables, creates an environment more favorable to the growth of latent tumors that then risk turning into cancer. Conversely, if the diet is rich in protective foods and contains only a small proportion of bad foods, microtumors cannot grow big enough, and the risk of developing cancer is lower (Figure 27).

There are many advantages to making the most of this long latency period for fighting cancer and thus effectively preventing its development with the help of the anticancer compounds in plants (Figure 28). From a strictly quantitative point of view, it is much easier to eliminate a few thousand cells in a benign microtumor than the billions of cancer cells that make up a mature tumor. For example, a highly effective anticancer molecule able to eliminate 99.9 percent of cancer cells could successfully eradicate a microtumor, whereas, in the case of a more advanced tumor, a number of cancer cells would likely survive this treatment. This effectiveness is all the greater since precancerous cells are at a vulnerable stage; as a result, they are much less able to modify their genes (mutation) in order to form the blood vessel network required for their energy needs and to create proteins that will enable them to resist the action of the anticancer molecules. In other words, the smaller and more immature the tumor, the better the chances of eliminating it.

## Looking for anticancer foods

Clearly, identifying food with significant amounts of anticancer molecules is of enormous importance for maximizing our chances of thwarting cancer. A well-established procedure consists of producing raw vegetable extracts, sterilizing the resulting mixtures and using this material to determine the degree to which they inhibit the growth of various tumors of human origin using cancer cell models cultivated in a laboratory (Figure 29). As an example, adding extracts of garlic, beet and some cabbages, like kale, is seen to stop the growth of cancer cells taken from breast and prostate tumors (Figure 30).

Some foods of plant origin also possess potent anti-inflammatory properties and can help prevent the creation of a climate of chronic inflammation favorable to cancer development. For example, the curcumin in turmeric and the resveratrol

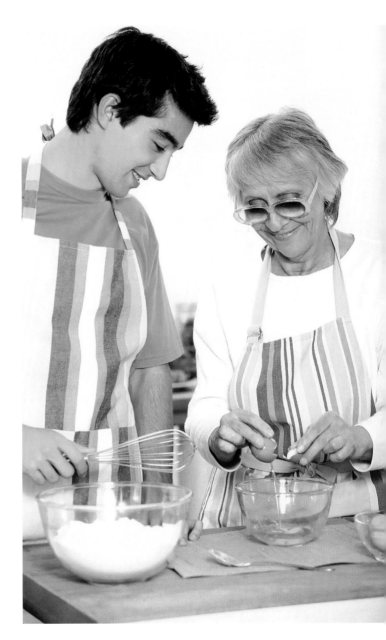

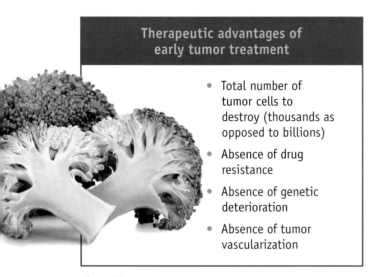

## Therapeutic advantages of early tumor treatment

- Total number of tumor cells to destroy (thousands as opposed to billions)
- Absence of drug resistance
- Absence of genetic deterioration
- Absence of tumor vascularization

**Figure 29**

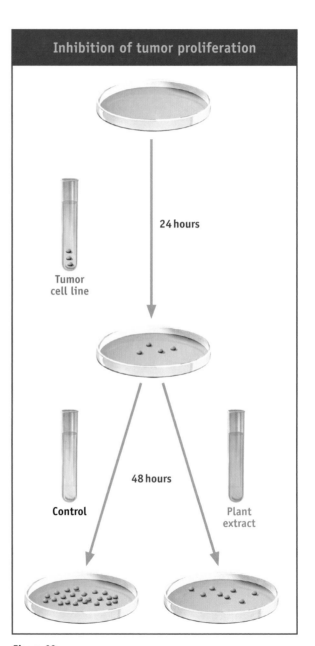

## Inhibition of tumor proliferation

24 hours

Tumor cell line

48 hours

Control

Plant extract

**Figure 28**

in red wine (see chapters 9 and 15) contain molecules capable of blocking a crucial step in the synthesis of COX-2 by cancer cells; this property plays an important role in their potential to interfere with the growth of some types of cancer cells. This anti-inflammatory property seems to be shared by many plants. In fact, research done in our laboratory indicates that adding gooseberry, blackberry or cranberry extracts to cells derived from a cancer of the prostate strikingly inhibits the increase in COX-2 caused by TNF, a powerful molecule involved in causing inflammation (Figure 31). Given the important role of inflammation in cancer development, it goes

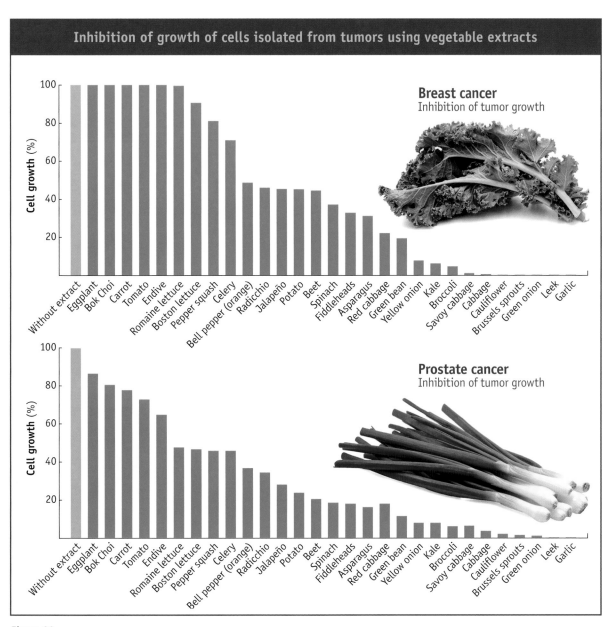

Figure 30

without saying that the anti-inflammatory properties of many foods cannot help but have an impact on cancer prevention.

All things considered, the lower incidence of cancer in individuals who eat the largest amounts of plants is directly linked to their anticancer compound content, which makes it possible to limit the development of microtumors developing spontaneously in our tissues. A constant dietary intake of these anticancer compounds forms the basis of any strategy aiming to prevent cancer development.

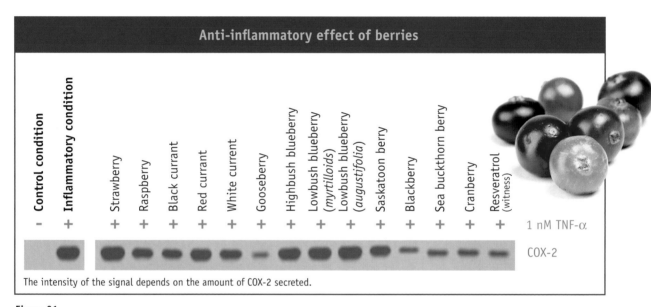

**Anti-inflammatory effect of berries**

The intensity of the signal depends on the amount of COX-2 secreted.

**Figure 31**

**In summary:**

- The foods selected during evolution contain beneficial compounds with anticancer properties in many ways similar to those of synthetic origin.

- Incorporating these compounds into the daily diet creates hostile conditions preventing the development of microtumor sites generated spontaneously during our lifetime.

- Preventing cancer through diet is equivalent to nontoxic chemotherapy, using anticancer molecules in foods that fight cancer at the source before it reaches maturity and threatens the proper functioning of the body.

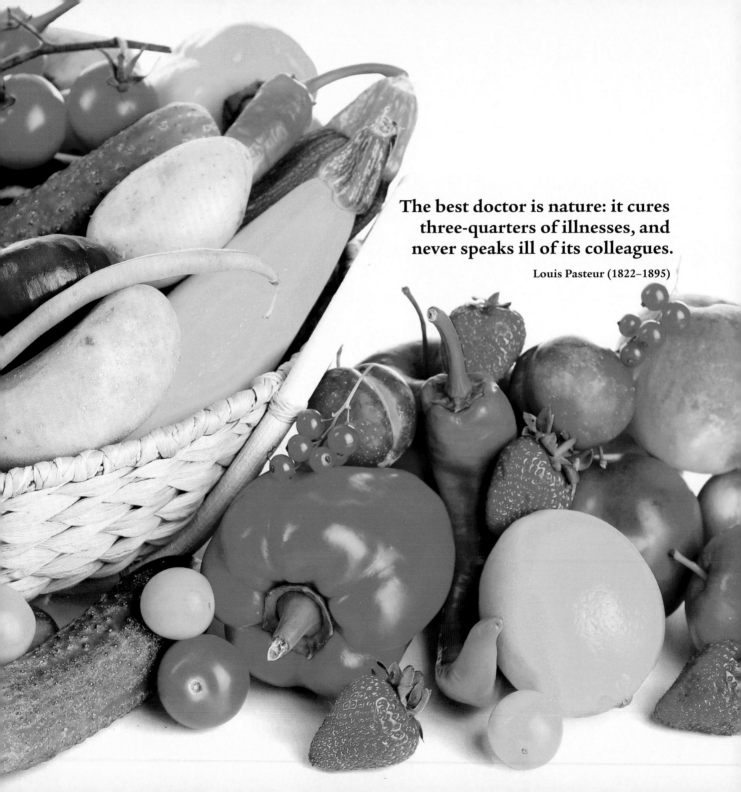

The best doctor is nature: it cures
three-quarters of illnesses, and
never speaks ill of its colleagues.

Louis Pasteur (1822–1895)

# Chapter 5

# Phytochemicals: An Anticancer Cocktail on Your Dinner Plate!

In nutrition, the foods we eat are generally considered from two angles. We talk about macronutrients (carbohydrates, proteins and fats) and micronutrients (vitamins and minerals) (Figure 32). This description is, however, incomplete, for in the case of fruits and vegetables their composition is not limited to nutrients. There is, in fact, another class of molecules found in significant amounts: phytochemical compounds (from the Greek *phyto*, meaning plant). These compounds are the molecules responsible for the color and organoleptic properties (affecting the sense organs) not only of fruits and vegetables, but also of many drinks and spices closely associated with the culinary traditions of many countries.

Raspberries' bright red color, garlic's typical odor or the strong astringent sensation caused by cocoa or tea are all characteristics directly linked to the various phytochemical compounds in these foods. And these compounds are very plentiful: a balanced diet including an array of fruits, vegetables and beverages like tea and red wine contains roughly 1 g to 2 g of phytochemical compounds, which is the same as ingesting a cocktail of approximately 5,000 to 10,000 different compounds a day! Far from being insignificant, the phytochemical content of fruits and vegetables is thus, without question, an essential characteristic of these foods (Figure 33).

Until very recently, vitamins, minerals and fiber were considered the only beneficial properties of fruits and vegetables for preventing chronic diseases, especially cancer. However, no study has yet shown that massive doses of vitamin supplements can supply any protection whatsoever against chronic diseases, including cancer. The results of many studies conducted on the subject actually indicate the opposite: there is an *increase* in risk of death associated with taking large doses of some of these supplements, especially beta-carotene, selenium, and vitamins A and E. From the point of view of cancer prevention, it is therefore more and more certain that the protection offered by regularly eating plant foods is primarily related to their phytochemical content.

## The phytochemical cocktail: An arsenal of anticancer molecules

Phytochemical compounds are the molecules that enable plants to defend themselves against infections and damage caused by microorganisms, insects and other predators.

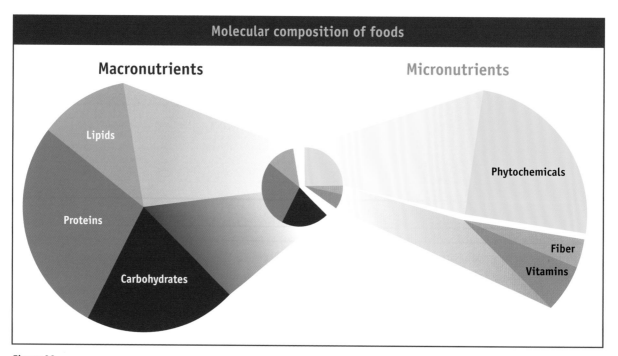

**Figure 32**

Plants cannot run away from their attackers and as a result have had to develop highly sophisticated protection systems to repel or counteract the harmful effects of attackers in their environment. These natural pesticides are essential for the survival of plant species and, in turn, all animals on the planet. Not to mention that several of these insecticides (caffeine, nicotine and morphine, among others) have a major influence on the daily lives of humankind due to their potent psychoactive properties!

The phytochemical compounds produced by plants have antibacterial, antifungal and insecticidal functions that reduce the harm caused by attackers and allow the plant to survive in hostile conditions. This is actually why these compounds are often found in large amounts in the parts most likely to be attacked by aggressors, notably the roots and fruits. For example, as we will see in Chapter 15, when grapes on the vine are attacked by certain microorganisms, they secrete large quantities of a substance that acts as a fungicide and counteracts the negative effect of these parasites.

The protective role of these various phytochemical compounds is not limited to their effects on plants' good health, however; these molecules also play a frontline role in our defense systems against cancer. Indeed, several studies of the compounds isolated from these foods have shown that a great many of them interfere with the various events involved in cancer development, and, as a result, could be *the most powerful weapon at our disposal to fight the development of this disease.*

For one thing, the tens of thousands of phytochemical compounds of plant origin have many pharmacological effects that hinder cancer progression, whether by directly attacking cancer cells, positively modulating the environment of these cells to keep them in a latent and harmless state or increasing the bioavailability of anticancer molecules (Figure 35).

Furthermore, plants have very low caloric density, and by eating them regularly, we can lower our energy intake and thus avoid gaining too much weight, a significant cancer risk factor. Nor should we ignore the major impact of foods of plant origin on the composition of intestinal bacterial flora: starches and fiber are not well absorbed by the intestine and are mostly fermented in

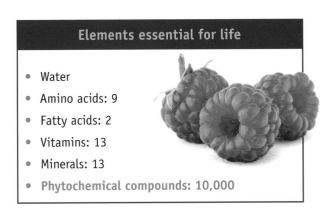

**Elements essential for life**

- Water
- Amino acids: 9
- Fatty acids: 2
- Vitamins: 13
- Minerals: 13
- **Phytochemical compounds: 10,000**

**Figure 33**

# Plant communication

Plants' amazing ability to defend themselves is clearly shown in the strategy used by the acacia. When kudus — a species of gazelle fond of the leaves of this tree — attack an acacia by grazing on its leaves, the tree reacts quickly by producing a gas, ethylene, that disperses in the air and reaches acacias located within a 165-foot (50 m) range. Upon contact with this gas, the trees produce tannins, astringent molecules that dry out the animal's mouth and discourage it from continuing to eat for long periods, which would devastate the foliage of the acacia population (Figure 34). Another tactic is used by some plants in response to damage caused by herbivorous insects like the American cricket (*Schistocerca americana*). During their "meal," these insects secrete a class of molecules, called caeliferins, that are rapidly recognized by the plant as a signal of the presence of an enemy. Plants then produce a very complex mixture of fragrant molecules that attract crickets' natural enemies and help them to get rid of their attackers. Although they are held prisoner by their roots and cannot move, plants nonetheless use their freedom of speech!

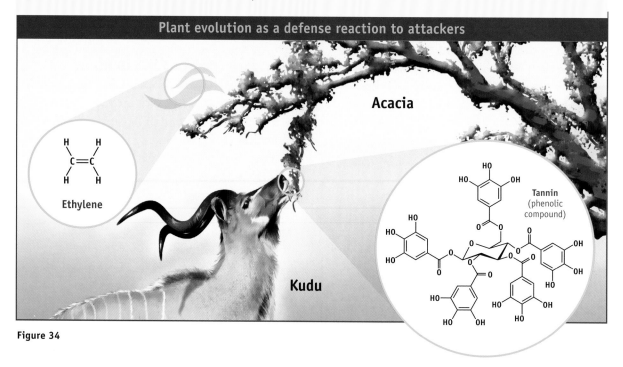

**Plant evolution as a defense reaction to attackers**

Acacia

Ethylene

Tannin
(phenolic compound)

Kudu

**Figure 34**

the colon by resident bacteria; this produces beneficial substances like short-chain fatty acids, with anti-inflammatory effects. This impact is important, because the composition of the intestinal flora, called the microbiome, is increasingly recognized as an essential component in the control of the metabolism and the prevention of chronic diseases in general. For example, the microbiome of obese people is different from that of slender people, and these differences have been associated with an increase in the risk of colon and liver cancers. It is interesting to note that some phytochemical compounds, especially polyphenols, are likewise very poorly absorbed by the intestine and also reach the colon, where they promote the growth of beneficial intestinal bacteria. Simply incorporating an abundance of plants into dietary habits thus encourages the establishment of a microbiome composed of an optimal proportion of beneficial bacteria essential for preventing cancer.

All plants contain many phytochemical compounds in varying amounts (Figure 36); they are what gives these foods their highly distinctive organoleptic properties (e.g., bitterness, astringency, smell). Some people's lack of enthusiasm for plants is related in large part to these organoleptic properties: whereas the taste of fats and sugar is immediately recognized by our brain as a synonym for a quick and efficient energy supply, the

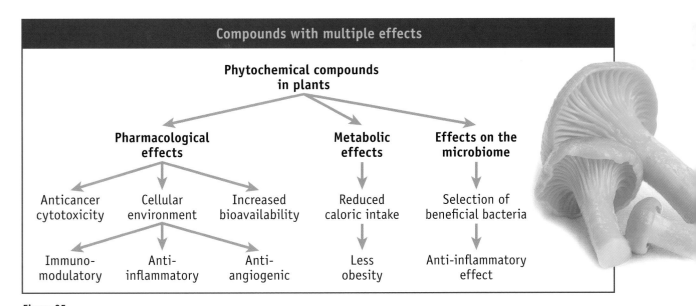

**Figure 35**

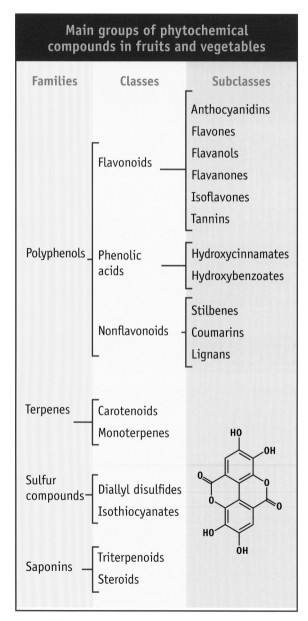

**Main groups of phytochemical compounds in fruits and vegetables**

| Families | Classes | Subclasses |
|---|---|---|
| Polyphenols | Flavonoids | Anthocyanidins |
| | | Flavones |
| | | Flavanols |
| | | Flavanones |
| | | Isoflavones |
| | | Tannins |
| | Phenolic acids | Hydroxycinnamates |
| | | Hydroxybenzoates |
| | Nonflavonoids | Stilbenes |
| | | Coumarins |
| | | Lignans |
| Terpenes | Carotenoids | |
| | Monoterpenes | |
| Sulfur compounds | Diallyl disulfides | |
| | Isothiocyanates | |
| Saponins | Triterpenoids | |
| | Steroids | |

**Figure 36**

bitterness and astringency of plants are instead interpreted as a potentially harmful attack. Fortunately, these reflexes in our primitive brain have gradually diminished during evolution, so that humans have been able to identify an ever-growing number of plant species that can actively contribute to maintaining good health.

The main phytochemical compounds in a food can often be very easily identified simply by its color or odor. For example, most brightly colored fruits are major sources of a class of molecules called polyphenols (Figure 37). More than 4,000 polyphenols have been identified to date, with these molecules being especially plentiful in some beverages like red wine and green tea, as well as in many solid foods like raisins, apples, onions and wild berries. They are also found in many herbs and spices, as well as in vegetables and nuts. Other classes of phytochemical compounds are instead characterized by their smell. For example, the smell of sulfur associated with crushed garlic or cooked cabbage is due to the sulfur compounds in these foods, whereas the odor (more pleasant) of citrus fruits is related to certain terpenes.

We will describe these various molecules in greater detail in the chapters devoted specifically to them, but we should start by saying that it is the high phytochemical content of some of the foods in these various classes that allows them to carry out their cancer-preventing functions and be considered nutraceuticals. In other words, a nutraceutical is a food, whether a fruit, vegetable, drink or fermented product, that contains in large amounts one or more molecules with anticancer potential.

The concept of nutraceuticals allows us to prioritize the choice of the foods we should include in a diet designed to prevent the development of cancer. For while all fruits and vegetables contain (by definition) phytochemical compounds, the *quantity* as well as the *nature* of these compounds varies widely from one fruit to another and one vegetable to another. All fruits and vegetables are not created equal: potatoes and carrots cannot be compared to broccoli and Savoy cabbage in terms of their cancer-fighting phytochemical content, any more than bananas can be compared to grapes or cranberries. There are significant differences in the levels of active compounds associated with foods and, in some cases, some compounds are only found in a single food.

These differences obviously have huge repercussions for cancer prevention: for example, when researchers examine the impact of total consumption of fruits and vegetables on cancer risk, they generally observe only a very slight decrease in risk, around 9 percent. On the other hand, when the consumption of certain specific plants is taken into account, the reduction in the risk for some cancers is

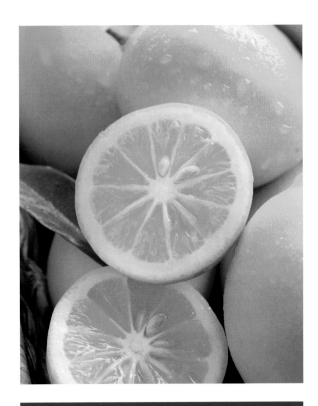

## Polyphenols and health

- Largest class of natural phytochemical compounds
- Molecules responsible for foods' astringency and bitterness
- Very wide variation in polyphenol intake depending on diet: from 0 g to 1 g per day

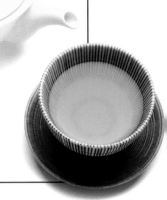

**Figure 37**

much greater. A study done on 76,000 women recently showed that those who regularly ate peaches and blueberries saw their risk of getting hormone-independent breast cancer decline by a third, whereas eating other fruits did not have a significant impact on risk (Figure 38). The same is observed for all plant foods: each class of foods is only active against certain specific cancers (Figure 39), and only by regularly eating a wide variety of plants with anticancer properties can these preventive activities be combined and the overall risk of cancer really be reduced.

This idea is key when trying to explain the anticancer properties of plants, since, coincidentally, many phytochemical compounds that show the greatest cancer-preventive activity are only found in certain very specific foods (Figure 40). The isoflavones in soy, the resveratrol in grapes, the curcumin in turmeric, the isothiocyanates and indoles in broccoli and the catechins in green tea are all anticancer molecules with an extremely limited distribution in nature. In other words, while it is true that, generally speaking, fruits and vegetables

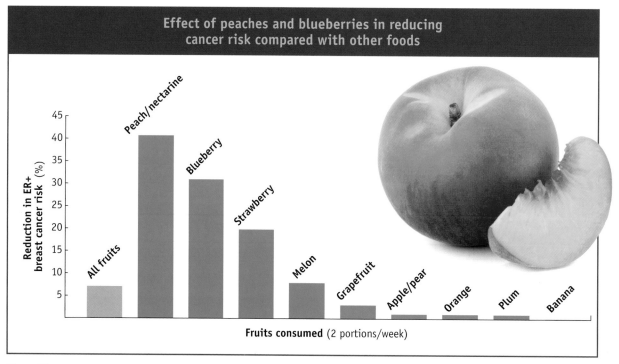

**Figure 38**

Adapted from Fung et al., 2013.

## Prospective studies showing the relationship between consuming specific foods and cancer incidence in human populations

| Food | Number of participants | Type of cancer | Reduction in risk (%) |
|---|---|---|---|
| Cruciferous vegetables | 47,909 | Bladder | 50 % |
| | 4,309 | Lung | 30 % |
| | 29,361 | Prostate | 50 % |
| Tomatoes | 47,365 | Prostate | 25 % |
| Citrus fruits | 521,457 | Stomach, esophagus | 25 % |
| | 477,312 | Stomach | 39 % |
| Green vegetables (dietary folate) | 81,922 | Pancreas | 75 % |
| | 11,699 | Breast (postmenopause) | 44 % |
| Green vegetables | 31,000 | Breast | 30 % |
| Lignans | 58,049 | Breast (ER+ postmenopause) | 28 % |
| Carrotes | 490,802 | Head and neck | 46 % |
| Apples, pears, plums | 490,802 | Head and neck | 38 % |
| Green tea | 69,710 | Colorectal | 57 % |
| Plant and nut oils (dietary tocopherol) | 295,344 | Prostate | 32 % |
| Vitamin D / calcium | 10,578 | Breast (postmenopause) | 35 % |
| Blueberries | 75,929 | Breast (ER-) | 31 % |
| Nuts | 75,680 | Pancreas | 35 % |

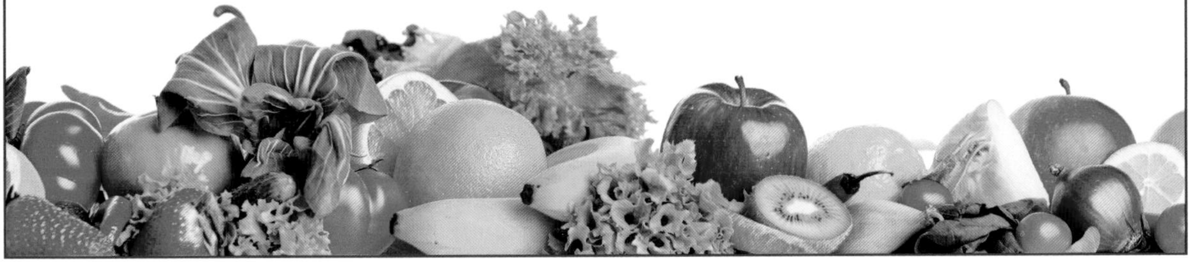

Figure 39

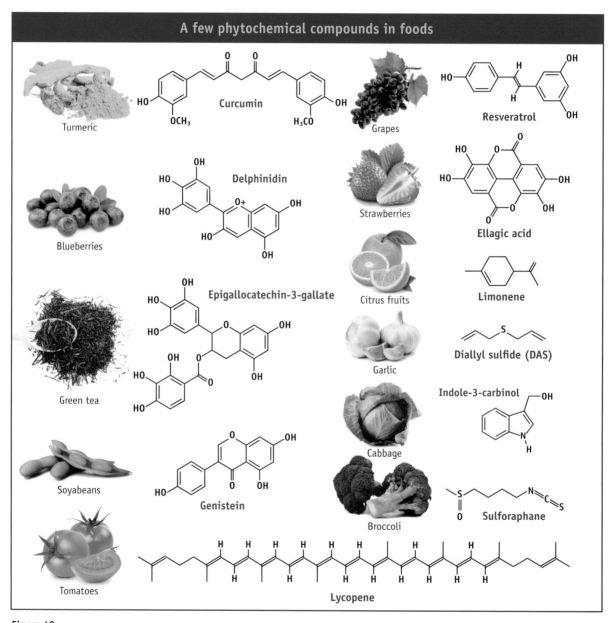

**A few phytochemical compounds in foods**

Turmeric — Curcumin

Grapes — Resveratrol

Blueberries — Delphinidin

Strawberries — Ellagic acid

Green tea — Epigallocatechin-3-gallate

Citrus fruits — Limonene

Garlic — Diallyl sulfide (DAS)

Cabbage — Indole-3-carbinol

Soyabeans — Genistein

Broccoli — Sulforaphane

Tomatoes — Lycopene

Figure 40

are an integral part of a balanced diet, the phytochemical compounds they contain must be examined more closely in the context of a diet aiming to reduce cancer risk.

Likewise, the scope of these recommendations must be broadened to include three foods among those with the highest levels of anticancer compounds found in nature — green tea, soy and turmeric. This is because, in addition to the scientific facts that unquestionably highlight the anticancer properties of the molecules in these foods, which we will discuss in the following chapters, we must point out a coincidence that speaks volumes: in countries with the lowest cancer rates, Asian countries in particular, green tea, soy and turmeric are fundamental elements in the diet.

This implies a need to considerably change the diet typical of Western countries. Combining foods as diverse as tomatoes, cabbage, green tea, peppers, turmeric, soy, garlic and grapes is in a way equivalent to incorporating thousands of years of culinary traditions developed by world cultures, both European and Asian. This is now possible for the vast majority of people, thanks to easy access to foodstuffs from the four corners of the earth.

## And much more than antioxidants!

Before describing the ways in which phytochemical compounds can help prevent cancer, a fundamental point must be mentioned: these molecules are not just antioxidants. It is impossible today to talk about the beneficial properties of a food without referring to its "antioxidant potential" or to its high "antioxidant" content. The term *antioxidant* is now so overused in the mass media that we might think that foods' only function is as a source of antioxidants (and obviously vitamins, but since most of the time vitamins have antioxidant properties…) and that it is this characteristic alone that makes a food good or bad for health (see box, p. 84).

True, several phytochemical compounds, especially polyphenols, have a chemical structure that is ideal for absorbing free radicals and these molecules are actually much more powerful antioxidants than vitamins are. For example, a medium apple, which contains relatively little vitamin C, about 10 mg, has antioxidant activity equivalent to that of 2,250 mg of vitamin C! In other words, the antioxidant properties of fruits and vegetables really stem from phytochemical compounds like polyphenols, with their vitamin content playing only a fairly minor role.

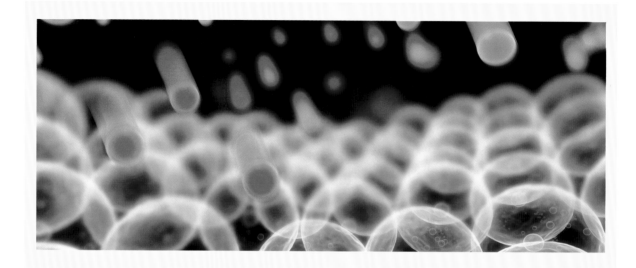

## What is an antioxidant?

The oxygen in the air we breathe provides fuel for our cells to produce biochemical energy in the form of an extremely important molecule, ATP. This combustion is not perfect, however, and generates considerable amounts of "waste products," commonly called "free radicals." These free radicals are harmful to cells, since they attack the structure of some cell components, especially DNA, proteins and lipids, causing considerable damage. As it ages, a cell can accumulate more than 50,000 lesions induced by free radicals, and this DNA deterioration may contribute to cancer (Figure 41).

To make it simpler, let's say that an antioxidant is simply a molecule that changes free radicals into harmless products, thereby reducing their damaging effects. Our cells contain several antioxidant molecules that protect themselves against free radicals, but this defense is likely insufficient to counter the negative effects of the multitude of toxic dietary and environmental agents all around us (e.g., ionizing radiation, ultraviolet rays, cigarette smoke). Adding antioxidants to the diet might therefore supply reinforcements to our cells' natural defense system and thus protect us from cancer. However, several studies have shown that antioxidant supplements (beta-carotene and vitamins A and E) have no effect on cancer risk and may even increase the risk of getting the disease.

On the other hand, other classes of compounds whose importance we will see in the next chapter, the isothiocyanates, have very average antioxidant activity and are nonetheless among the molecules with the greatest influence on cancer development. So, while antioxidant activity is a *property* of many molecules, this property is not necessarily what causes its biological effects. Antioxidant theory is more or less consistent with certain data accumulated over time; thus, while a baked potato (with its skin) has an antioxidant activity four times higher than broccoli, 12 times higher than cauliflower and 25 times higher than carrots, it shows little potential for preventing cancer. As a result, while antioxidant properties are a common characteristic of many foods of plant origin and may certainly help counteract the harmful effects of free radicals, especially where the oxidation of blood vessel walls at the root of several cardiovascular diseases is concerned, we must nonetheless stop seeing these foods only as sources of antioxidants. This is why the United States Department of Agriculture (USDA) recently stopped publishing data on the antioxidant activity of various foods, to prevent manufacturers from distorting these figures to promote the benefits of their products.

On the contrary, the advantage of a diet based on a daily intake of nutraceuticals lies in the great versatility in the mode of action of the compounds in these foods. Far from just being free radical neutralizers, phytochemical compounds have the property of targeting a large number of distinct events, all related to cancer development (Figure 42), with some of these molecules acting on several levels. Active compounds like those in garlic and cabbage prevent the activation of carcinogenic substances, while others, like some polyphenols (resveratrol, curcumin, catechins or genistein), prevent tumor growth by interfering directly with tumor cells or by halting the formation of new blood vessels necessary for cancer development. In several ways, the processes targeted by compounds of nutritional origin are analogous to those of

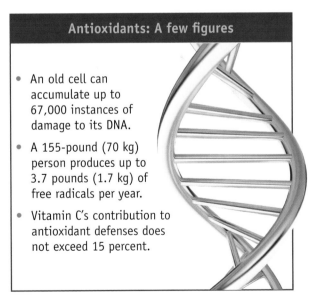

**Antioxidants: A few figures**

- An old cell can accumulate up to 67,000 instances of damage to its DNA.

- A 155-pound (70 kg) person produces up to 3.7 pounds (1.7 kg) of free radicals per year.

- Vitamin C's contribution to antioxidant defenses does not exceed 15 percent.

**Figure 41**

synthetic molecules currently being developed as drugs, illustrating yet again the degree to which foods high in anticancer molecules possess an action similar to that of drugs. This combination of phytochemical compounds thus gives the tumor very little chance to develop, for by eliminating the mutagenic activity of carcinogens right from the start, and by controlling the growth of microscopic tumors that have managed to develop in spite of everything, these compounds keep the eventual tumor in a primitive state that will not damage the organism.

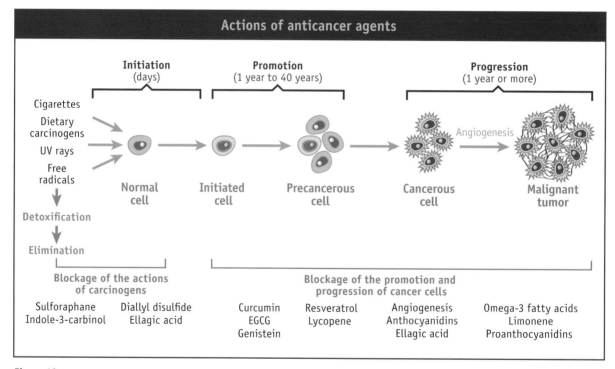

Figure 42

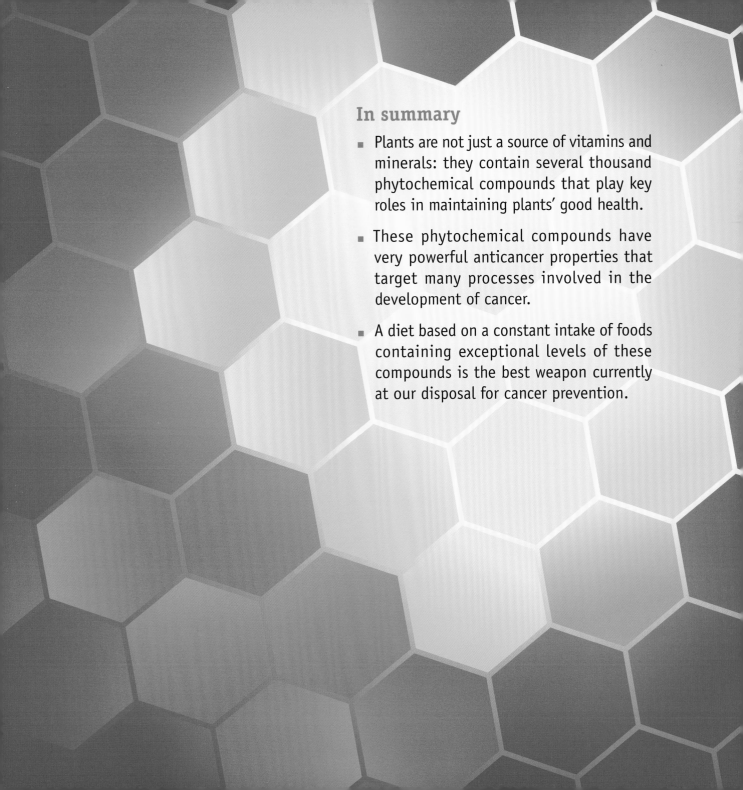

## In summary

- Plants are not just a source of vitamins and minerals: they contain several thousand phytochemical compounds that play key roles in maintaining plants' good health.

- These phytochemical compounds have very powerful anticancer properties that target many processes involved in the development of cancer.

- A diet based on a constant intake of foods containing exceptional levels of these compounds is the best weapon currently at our disposal for cancer prevention.

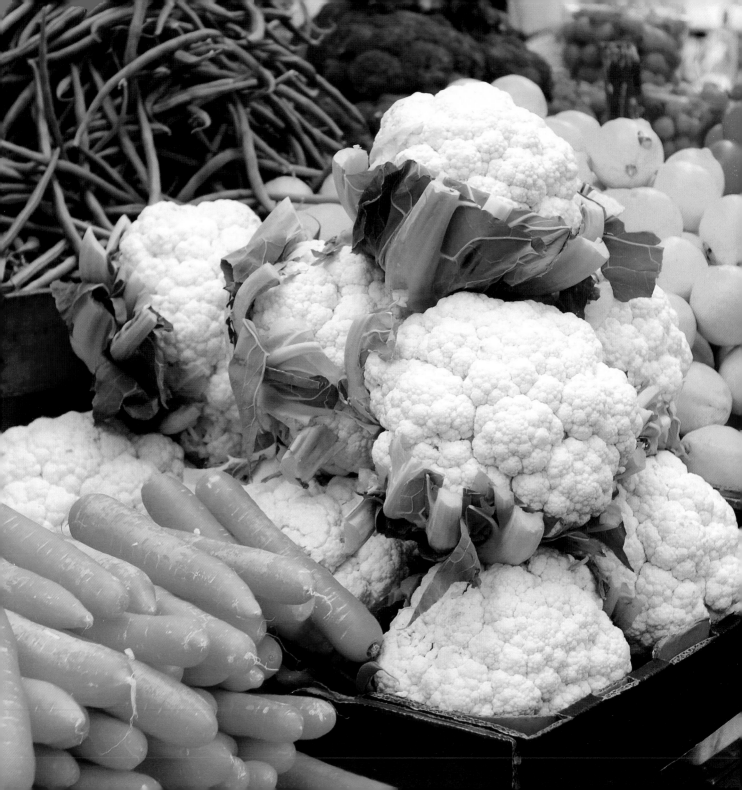

# Part II

# Foods that fight cancer

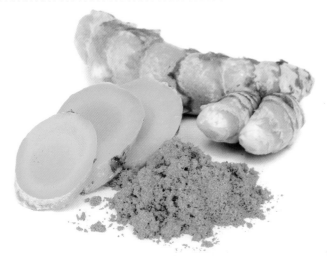

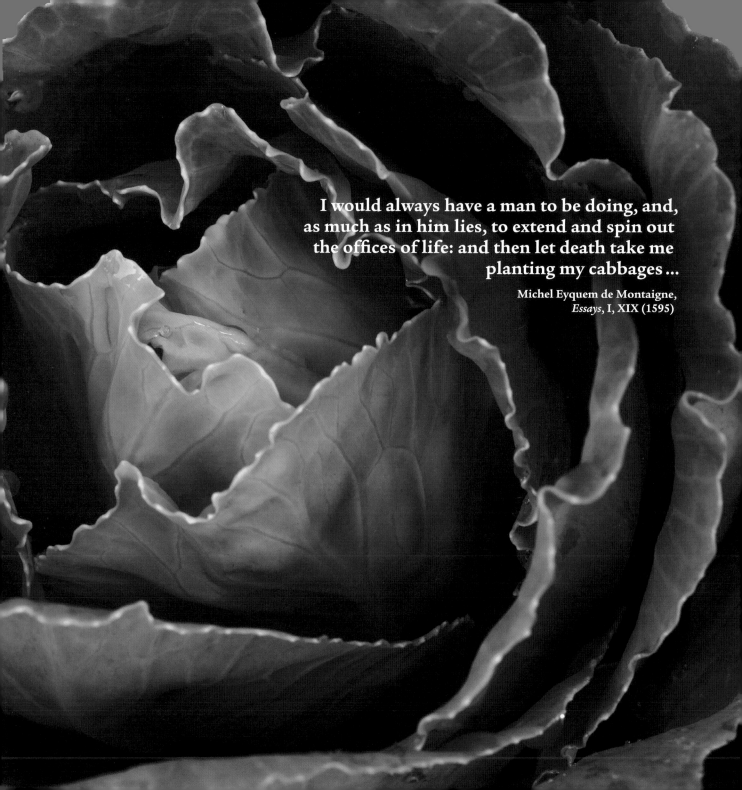

I would always have a man to be doing, and, as much as in him lies, to extend and spin out the offices of life: and then let death take me planting my cabbages...

Michel Eyquem de Montaigne, *Essays*, I, XIX (1595)

# Chapter 6

# Cancer Cells Hate Cabbage

A Greek legend based on the tales in *The Iliad* claims that Dionysus, the god of the grape harvest, was very badly received on his way through Thrace. The warlike Lycurgus, King of the Edonians, beat back the god's army using his cattle-prod, forcing him to take refuge in the grotto of Thetis, the sea nymph. However, driven mad by this victory, Lycurgus began to destroy what he thought were the god's sacred vines, but which were in fact the feet of his own son, Dryas. Dionysus punished the king for this sacrilege by bringing a terrible drought on the Thracian people, and his anger could only be appeased by putting Lycurgus to death. Tortured and dismembered by the Edonians, Lycurgus wept in pain before dying, and where his tears fell, there sprouted cabbages.

Far from being the only fanciful story associated with cabbage (just think of its role in the birth of babies), this legend nonetheless reflects the important role played by this vegetable in the history of European and Mediterranean civilizations. Cultivated for more than 6,000 years, and as a result likely the elder statesman of our vegetables, cabbage is found everywhere, both in the history of food and in ancient and medieval literary traditions; and, as Rabelais said in the adventures of Pantagruel, "O thrice and four times happy those who plant cabbages," since its cultivation was a symbol of tranquility and pacifism.

However, these vegetables are not among the foods that arouse the most passion and

*(Continued on page 94)*

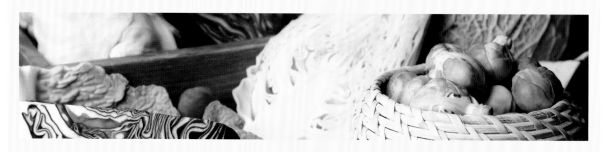

## Cabbages

Plants in the cabbage family belong to a subfamily of crucifers known botanically by the name *Brassica*. The main cabbages consumed, all descendants of the *Brassica oleracea* species, are white or green "headed" cabbage (*B. o. capitata*), broccoli (*B. o. italic*), cauliflower (*B. o. botrytis*), brussels sprouts (*B. o. gemmifera*) and leafy cabbage greens (*B. o. acephala*) like kale and collards. The edible Asian cabbages are the descendants of a different *Brassica* species with a more delicate flavor. At one time there were hundreds of distinct varieties of cabbage that have now disappeared, likely due to commercial pressures for uniformity and productivity. Note that turnips, mustard, cress, arugula and radishes are also cruciferous vegetables, as are the oleaginous species of rapeseed and its Canadian cultivar, canola.

### Cabbage

This category includes various cabbages that are distinctive in both shape and color: white or red smooth-leaved cabbage, as well as green Milanese cabbage (Savoy cabbage), with crinkly or curly leaves; this is often called kale in North America, but is not to be confused with European kale, a leafy non-head-forming cabbage.

### Broccoli

Now a star vegetable in any "healthy" diet worthy of the name, for a long time broccoli was actually relatively unknown outside its countries of origin, southern Italy and Greece. The word "broccoli" is derived from the Latin *bracchium*, meaning "branch," probably because of its bouquetlike shape, similar to that of a small tree. Broccoli growing was long limited to Italy, and then to the eastern Mediterranean, following the decline of the Roman Empire. It was not until the marriage of Catherine de Medici and Henry II, at the beginning of the

16th century, that it appeared in France under the name "Italian asparagus." Similarly, it was only with the large-scale arrival of Italian immigrants that broccoli made its appearance in North America, where it is now one of the most popular green vegetables.

## Cauliflower

*Cauli-flori* to the Romans, Syrian cabbage to the 12th-century Arabs, this variety of cabbage is likely a descendant of broccoli that migrated toward the Middle East after the fall of the Roman Empire and later returned to Europe. "Cauliflower is nothing but cabbage with a college education," wrote Mark Twain ironically in *The Tragedy of Pudd'nhead Wilson,* and he was perhaps not wrong, when we consider the considerable efforts that were necessary to select this cabbage, with its abundant flowers and lack of chlorophyll, a result of their being enveloped in a thick layer of leaves.

## Brussels sprouts

It could almost be said that the world is divided in two: those who like brussels sprouts and those who can't stand them. It is thought that this species of cabbage appeared in the 13th century, but it only really developed after the beginning of the 18th century in northern Europe, near brussels, quite simply in order to get the maximum benefit from the arable land needed to supply the city's ever-growing population. It was a success on all fronts, judging by the 20 to 40 little cabbages that grow on a single stem. Brussels sprouts are really in a class of their own in terms of their anticancer phytochemical compound contents and, if they are not overcooked, they can play a worthy role in a cancer prevention strategy.

## "Leafy" cabbage

This cabbage of the *acephala* variety, which literally means "headless," is characterized by thick, flat leaves, relatively smooth in the case of collards or very curly in the case of kale. Botanists consider that these cabbages, and especially kale, are probably closest in shape to the original wild cabbage, and thus that these species are certainly among the first cultivated cabbages. What's more, the father of botany, the Greek Theophrastus (372–287 BCE), lists in his treatises the growing of several species of cabbage, including kale, later confirmed by the Romans Pliny and Cato. Especially popular in northern Europe, these cabbages deserve to be better known, as they are exceptional sources of iron, vitamins A and C, folic acid and anticancer compounds, as we will see later.

enthusiasm in people, to say the least! Tasteless to some, lacking in delicacy to others, cabbage and its cousins are to a greater or lesser degree disliked by some people. Yet, harvested at the right time and prepared properly, they can be a real treat, especially since they are among the foods with the greatest ability to effectively ward off the development of cancer.

Cabbage is the prototype of a family of vegetables called *crucifers*, a term that describes the cross shape of the flowers the plant produces in order to reproduce. Even though it may at first be hard to believe, the main species of cabbage found today — broccoli, cauliflower, brussels sprouts, kale, etc. — are all direct descendants of wild cabbage (see box, pp. 92–93). From this plant (*Brassica oleracea*), which still grows wild on the rugged terrain of the rocky hills and cliffs of the Atlantic coast of Europe and the Mediterranean, humans domesticated cabbage and forced evolution's hand by selecting, about 4,000 years ago, specimens with very specific characteristics satisfying the culinary tastes of peoples in the region. For example, the Romans seemed to prefer a cabbage with massive flowers and succeeded in developing the first varieties of broccoli and, later on, cauliflower. The diversification of the *Brassica* species must have been an extremely important activity in antiquity, for specialists believe that most species of cabbage now known already existed in the Roman era, three centuries BCE.

## The therapeutic qualities of cabbage

In ancient times, it seems that plants in the crucifer family were mainly grown for their medicinal qualities. Beginning with mustard, cultivated in China more than 6,000 years ago, and followed by the various forms of cabbage described by Greek and Roman botanists, cultivation basically aimed to produce plants to treat various disorders, from deafness to gout, as well as gastrointestinal problems. Cabbage, in particular, was considered to be a very important medicinal food for the Greek and Roman civilizations, even replacing garlic, at one point, as the favorite remedy. Praised by Pythagoras, baptized "the vegetable of a thousand virtues" by Hippocrates (460–377 BCE), who recommended it as a cure for diarrhea and dysentery, among other things, cabbage was considered at the time to be a food necessary for good health. And rightly so, since Diogenes the Cynic (413–327 BCE) lived to the venerable age of 83, having only a poor barrel as his dwelling and eating almost nothing but cabbage.

Marcus Porcius Cato, or Cato the Elder (234–149 BCE), a very powerful Roman statesman who occupied the most honorable and most feared of all posts — that of censor, the magistrate notably responsible for establishing tax amounts — was the first to use the term *Brassica* (from the Celtic *bresic*, meaning "cabbage"), still used today to designate the vegetables in this family. Highly suspicious of doctors, all of whom were Greeks at the time, Cato viewed cabbage as a universal remedy for diseases, a true fountain of youth responsible for his good health and virility (he had a son at age 80). While he filled his leisure time by growing more than a hundred medicinal plants, Cato wrote in his treatise on agriculture *De agri cultura* that "eaten raw with vinegar, cooked in oil or fat, cabbage eliminates everything and cures everything," from a hangover caused by too much wine to a number of serious illnesses; according to him, applying a crushed cabbage leaf soothed ulcers on the breasts. While luckily we now have more effective modern means to treat breast cancer, the role of cabbage as a cure for overindulgence in alcohol seems to have come down through the ages, judging by the recent appearance on the Russian market of a salty beverage made from cabbage juice and designed to alleviate those unpleasant post-celebration aftereffects.

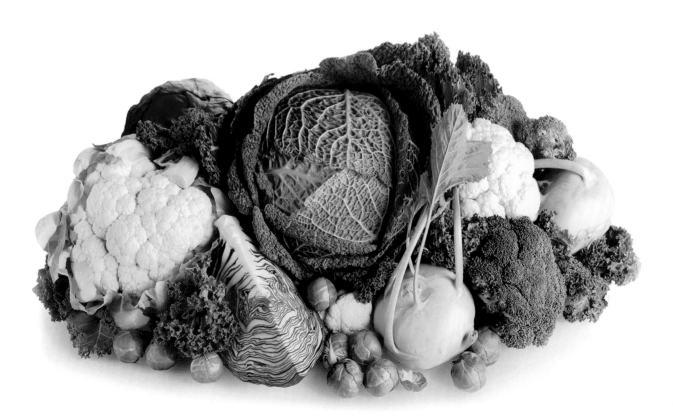

## The anticancer effects of cruciferous vegetables

Studies done to date indicate that cruciferous vegetables are among the main sources of the anticancer properties associated with the consumption of fruits and vegetables. For example, in the course of a study analyzing 252 cases of bladder cancer in 47,909 health professionals over a period of 10 years, eating five or more servings of cruciferous vegetables a week, especially broccoli or cabbage, was associated with cutting the risk of bladder cancer in half, compared with individuals who only ate one serving or less of these vegetables. The observation was the same for breast cancer: Swedish women who ate the most crucifers, one or two servings a day, saw their risk of developing breast cancer cut in half compared with those who ate none or few. Without listing all of the studies suggesting that cruciferous vegetables have a real chemoprotective effect, it must be mentioned that eating them regularly has also been associated with a lower risk of several other cancers, like those of the lung, the gastrointestinal system (stomach, colon, rectum) and the prostate (Figure 43). In the latter case, three or more servings of cruciferous vegetables a week have even been shown to be more effective in preventing prostate cancer than eating tomatoes, often suggested as a food that prevents the development of this disease (see Chapter 13).

A protective effect of crucifers is also observed in the prevention of recurrences in people with some types of cancer (secondary prevention). For example, patients with bladder cancer who eat at least one serving of broccoli a week see their risk of mortality linked to this cancer decrease by 60 percent. In the same vein, studies indicate that breast

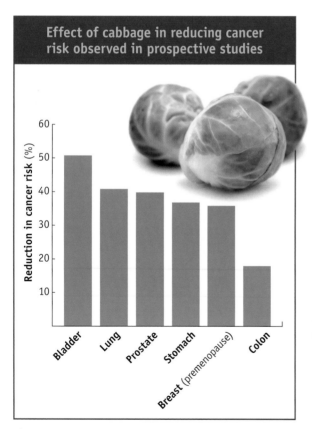

**Effect of cabbage in reducing cancer risk observed in prospective studies**

Reduction in cancer risk (%)

Bladder — Lung — Prostate — Stomach — Breast (premenopause) — Colon

**Figure 43**

cancer survivors who eat three servings of crucifers weekly have a 50 percent lower risk of recurrence.

So, while the quantity of fruits and vegetables in the diet definitely plays a key role in preventing cancer, the data indicate that some kinds of vegetables, especially crucifers, are particularly important for halting the development of the disease. These observations are critical in the context of the Western diet, and especially the North American diet, where potatoes make up as much as 50 percent of daily fruit and vegetable intake and cruciferous vegetables still play only a very limited role.

| Glucosinolate content in the main cruciferous vegetables | |
| --- | --- |
| Cruciferous vegetables | Glucosinolates (mg/100 g) |
| Brussels sprouts | 237 |
| Collards | 201 |
| Kale | 101 |
| Watercress | 95 |
| Turnip | 93 |
| Cabbage (white or red) | 65 |
| Broccoli | 62 |
| Cauliflower | 43 |
| Chinese cabbage (bok choi) | 54 |
| Chinese cabbage (pe-tsaï) | 21 |

**Figure 44**    Adapted from McNaughton and Marks, 2003. The amounts indicated are an average of results obtained to date.

## Phytochemical compounds in vegetables in the cabbage family

The dramatic effects of vegetables in the cabbage family on the decrease in risk of developing several cancers suggest that these vegetables are a significant source of phytochemical compounds. Of all the plants eaten by humans, cruciferous vegetables are probably those that contain the greatest variety of phytochemical molecules with anticancer properties. In addition to several polyphenols found in other protective foods, discussed later, cruciferous vegetables also contain a group of compounds called *glucosinolates* (Figure 44). These molecules are especially plentiful in brussels sprouts and leafy cabbages (kale and collards), but they are also found in significant amounts in all crucifers.

## Glucosinolates

Contrary to most of the phytochemical compounds we will describe in the following chapters, the importance of glucosinolates in cancer prevention through food is not directly linked to these molecules; they work instead by releasing two classes of compounds with very powerful anticancer activity, *isothiocyanates* and *indoles*.

## Cruciferous vegetables: Isothiocyanates

| Vegetables | Main isothiocyanates |
|---|---|
| Cabbage | Allyl isothiocyanate |
| | 3-Methylsulfinylpropyl isothiocyanate |
| | 4-Methylsulfinylbutyl isothiocyanate |
| | 3-Methylthiopropyl isothiocyanate |
| | 4-Methylthiobutyl isothiocyanate |
| | 2-Phenylethyl isothiocyanate |
| | Benzyl isothiocyanate |
| Broccoli | Sulforaphane |
| | 3-Methylsulfinylpropyl isothiocyanate |
| | 3-Butenyl isothiocyanate |
| | Allyl isothiocyanate |
| | 4-Methylsulfinylbutyl isothiocyanate |
| Turnip | 2-Phenylethyl isothiocyanate |
| Watercress | 2-Phenylethyl isothiocyanate |
| Garden cress | Benzyl isothiocyanate |
| Radish | 4-Methylthio-3-butenyl isothiocyanate |

Figure 45

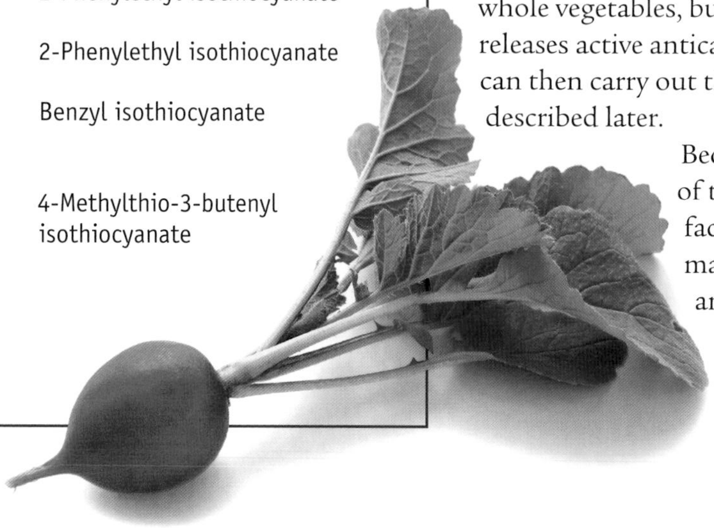

Over a hundred glucosinolates occur in nature, acting as a "reservoir" for storing many different isothiocyanates and indoles, all with very high anticancer potential (Figure 45). When the vegetable is chewed, the plant cells are crushed, which mixes up the various compartments in the cells that are usually separated from each other.

Glucosinolates that were stored in one of the compartments of broccoli cells are thus exposed to *myrosinase*, an enzyme found in another compartment whose role is to cleave off some parts of the glucosinolate molecules. When broccoli is chewed, the vegetable's main isothiocyanate, glucoraphanin, suddenly finds itself in the presence of myrosinase and is immediately turned into sulforaphane, a powerful anticancer molecule (Figure 46). To put it another way, the anticancer molecules in cruciferous vegetables occur in a latent state in whole vegetables, but eating these vegetables releases active anticancer compounds that can then carry out the anticancer functions described later.

Because of the complexity of this mechanism, several factors must be considered to maximize the isothiocyanate and indole intake offered by this cruciferous vegetable. First of all, it is important to note that glucosinolates are very soluble in water: cooking crucifers in a large volume of water for just 10 minutes reduces the quantity of glucosinolates in these vegetables by half and should therefore be avoided. Secondly, myrosinase activity is very sensitive to heat, so that prolonged cooking of vegetables, whether or not in a large volume of water, substantially reduces the quantity of isothiocyanates that can be released when the vegetable is eaten. Studies suggest that some of the bacteria in the intestinal flora might change glucosinolates into isothiocyanates and thus make up for the inactivation of the vegetable caused by heat, but such a role still has to be clearly established. Cruciferous vegetables should therefore be cooked as little as possible, in a minimum of water, to reduce the loss of myrosinase and glucosinolate activity caused

by immersing these vegetables in water. Quick-cooking techniques like steaming or stir-frying in a wok are definitely easy ways to maximize the quantity of anticancer molecules supplied by cruciferous vegetables, as well as making these vegetables generally more attractive and tasty. Frozen products go through a high-temperature blanching stage during processing, which reduces both their glucosinolate content and their myrosinase activity; as a result, these products are definitely inferior to fresh vegetables as a source of anticancer molecules. Lastly, to promote the release of active molecules, remember to chew your vegetables well before swallowing!

## Sulforaphane, the "star" of the isothiocyanates

Isothiocyanates contain in their structure an atom of sulfur, the main cause of the characteristic odor produced by overcooking cabbages and their cousins. Since each isothiocyanate is derived from a different glucosinolate, the nature of the isothiocyanates associated with cruciferous vegetables obviously depends on the nature of the glucosinolates in these vegetables. Some glucosinolates are found in almost all cruciferous vegetables, whereas other members of this family contain very high levels of a specific type of glucosinolate, and

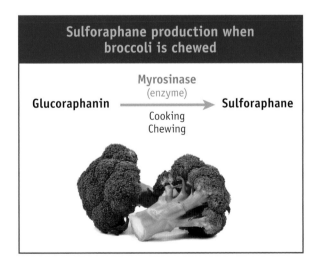

**Figure 46**

therefore of the corresponding isothiocyanate. These differences in composition are important, since some isothiocyanates have more powerful anticancer properties than others. This is notably the case for the sulforaphane associated with broccoli.

Sulforaphane was isolated for the first time in 1959 from whitetop, or hoary cress (*Cardaria draba*), where it occurs in very large quantities. From a nutritional point of view, broccoli is by far the best source of sulforaphane, however, with up to 60 mg of this molecule per serving. It is also interesting to note that broccoli sprouts can contain up to 100 times more sulforaphane than mature broccoli.

Sulforaphane, and therefore broccoli, deserves special consideration in any dietary strategy for preventing cancer. This interest is justified by a number of results obtained

through research during the last 20 years indicating that sulforaphane considerably speeds up the body's elimination of toxic substances with the potential to cause cancer. This is significant, as increasing the effectiveness of detoxification systems by means of sulforaphane clearly reduces the occurrence, number and size of mammary tumors in rats and mice caused by certain carcinogenic substances. As we have already seen, epidemiological studies indicate that this anticancer effect applies equally to humans.

Sulforaphane also seems to be able to act directly on cancer cells and cause their death by triggering the apoptosis process. In a series of studies on the ability of substances of nutritional origin to cause the death of cells isolated from an infantile brain tumor, called a medullablastoma, we have observed that sulforaphane is the only molecule of nutritional origin tested able to cause cell death. The ability of sulforaphane to cause the death of cancer cells has also been observed for other kinds of tumors, such as cancers of the colon and prostate, as well as in the case of acute lymphoblastic leukemia, and therefore suggests that the direct action of the molecule on tumor cells contributes to its anticancer properties.

Sulforaphane also has bactericidal antibiotic properties, especially against *Helicobacter pylori*, the bacterium causing gastric ulcers. This

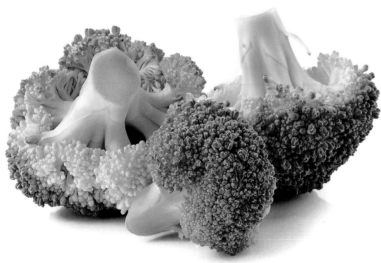

activity, at first glance not directly related to cancer, could nonetheless play a very important role in protecting against stomach cancer, since it is now thought that being infected with *H. pylori*, with the gastric ulcers that result, considerably increases (by three to six times) the risk of cancer in this organ. Eating broccoli would put sulforaphane into direct contact with the bacteria in the stomach itself and prevent the development of this disease at the source. All of these properties make sulforaphane the isothiocyanate with the most powerful anticancer potential and, in turn, make broccoli one of the most important foods for preventing the appearance of several cancers.

Despite all of the beneficial properties associated with sulforaphane, it would be incorrect to think that eating broccoli regularly can by itself help prevent cancer. The isothiocyanates and indoles occurring in other members of the crucifer family also have many anticancer properties that apparently contribute to the protective effect of these vegetables. Among these molecules, two deserve special attention: phenethyl isothiocyanate (PEITC) and indole-3-carbinol (I3C).

## PEITC

Phenethyl isothiocyanate (PEITC) is a molecule formed from gluconasturtiin, a glucosinolate found in large quantities in watercress and Chinese cabbage. Just like sulforaphane, PEITC can protect laboratory animals from cancers caused by exposure to toxic substances, especially cancers of the esophagus, stomach, colon and lung. In the latter case, some studies have shown that an increased intake of cress in the diet of a group of smokers (60 g per meal for three days) was associated with a decrease in the toxic forms of NNK, a carcinogenic nitrosamine in tobacco. Given the very strong carcinogenic potential of NNK, these results clearly illustrate the degree to which isothiocyanates act as powerful protective agents against the development of tumors caused by carcinogenic substances.

It seems more and more certain that PEITC's anticancer action mechanism might also involve direct action on cancer cells. PEITC is in fact one of the isothiocyanates most toxic for cancer cells, especially leukemia cells and those in colon, breast and prostate cancers, with this effect being linked to the molecule's ability to force the cells to die through apoptosis. This property suggests therefore that PEITC might not only prevent tumors from developing, but might also play a preventive role in the case of pre-existing tumors. Recent observations do indeed indicate that PEITC is able to eliminate cancer stem cells, a subpopulation of tumor cells that often resist anticancer treatments and are responsible for many recurrences.

These observations indicate that dietary sources of PEITC, like watercress, can therefore be an additional barrier against the development of certain types of cancer, both because of their ability to counteract the action of highly carcinogenic substances and because of their cytotoxic properties with respect to cancer cells.

## Indole-3-carbinol

Even though it is a product of the hydrolysis of glucosinolates, like isothiocyanates, I3C is different from this class of molecules, both in its chemical structure (without any sulfur atoms) and its anticancer mode of action. I3C is derived from the degradation of glucobrassicin, a glucosinolate found in the vast majority of cruciferous vegetables, although it is slightly more plentiful in broccoli and brussels sprouts.

More recent research into the chemopreventive role of I3C shows an impact on estrogen metabolism and its ability to interfere with estrogen-dependent cancers like those of the breast, endometrium and cervix. In fact, it seems like I3C has the ability to cause changes in the structure of estradiol that reduce this hormone's ability to encourage cell growth in these tissues.

This effect is clearly illustrated by results showing that cells in the cervix containing human papilloma virus (HPV) 16 (the main cause of this cancer) and able to develop into cancer cells after estrogen treatment see their growth halted by the administration of I3C.

In conclusion, the considerable efforts made by our far-off ancestors to produce all of these varieties of cabbage were certainly worth the trouble when we consider the exceptional phytochemical content of these cruciferous vegetables, especially glucosinolates and their active forms, isothiocyanates and indoles. Including these vegetables in the diet is thus an easy way to supply the body with generous amounts of these molecules and, as a result, prevent the development of several cancers, especially in the lungs and gastrointestinal tract. Currently available data are particularly encouraging. For example, a diet containing three or four servings of broccoli a week, which is far from excessive, has proven to be enough to protect people from colon polyps, a significant stage in the development of cancer in this organ. Finally, the inhibiting action of some components of crucifers on estrogen makes these vegetables essential players in the fight against breast cancer.

**In summary:**

- Cruciferous vegetables contain large quantities of several anticancer compounds that hinder the development of cancer by preventing carcinogenic substances from causing cell damage.

- Broccoli and brussels sprouts are exceptional sources of these anticancer molecules.

- Light cooking, as well as chewing the vegetables well, is necessary to get the most from their anticancer potential.

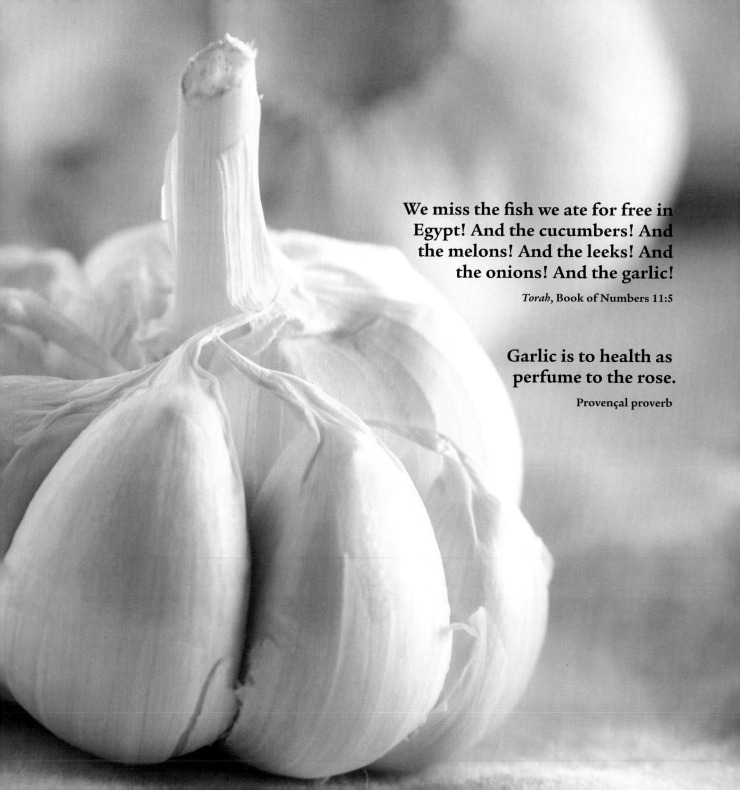

We miss the fish we ate for free in Egypt! And the cucumbers! And the melons! And the leeks! And the onions! And the garlic!

*Torah*, Book of Numbers 11:5

Garlic is to health as perfume to the rose.

Provençal proverb

# Chapter 7

# Garlic and Onions: Keeping Cancer at Bay

The many historical references to the use of garlic and its cousins in the *Allium* family (onion, leek, etc.) (see box, pp. 106–107) by ancient civilizations represent one of the best documented examples of plants being used to treat diseases and maintain overall health. Throughout the history of the greatest civilizations, garlic has always been considered both a food and a medicine and, as a result, no other plant family is as intrinsically linked to the blossoming of the world's culinary and medical cultures.

The cultivation of garlic and onions probably originated in Central Asia and the Middle East at least 5,000 years ago, and subsequently spread toward the Mediterranean, Egypt in particular, and to the Far East, where their use in cooking was already common in China more than 2,000 years BCE. The Egyptians were especially fond of garlic and onions, and attributed strength and endurance to them. In addition, the Greek historian Herodotus of Halicarnassus (484–425 BCE) tells in his writings of the discovery of inscriptions on the Great Pyramid of Cheops describing the considerable sum (1,600 silver talents) spent to feed the workers meals based on garlic and onions.

Far from being a food strictly for the working class, garlic held a very important

*(Continued on page 108)*

# The main members of the *Allium* family

## Garlic

Undoubtedly the most widespread condiment in the world, garlic (*Allium sativa*) is an essential ingredient in most culinary traditions. In Chinese writing, the word for "garlic," *suan*, is represented by a single character, implying that this food was already widely used at the beginning of the language's evolution. Used since antiquity to treat animal bites, such as snakebites, garlic even acquired the legendary reputation of being one of the most effective ways of scaring off vampires. This legend is all the more strange given that the anticoagulant properties associated with eating garlic should instead be attractive to such inveterate blood-drinkers!

## Onions

Native to Eurasia, the *Allium cepa* bulb is now grown and eaten as a vegetable and condiment all over the world. An essential part of Egyptian culture, where they were believed to possess the qualities of strength and power, a symbol of intelligence in ancient China and a staple vegetable in the medieval European diet, onions have long been integral to the culinary traditions of all civilizations. In terms of phytochemicals, onions are a major source of the flavonoid quercetin, containing as much as 50 mg per 100 g. The molecule that causes onions' tear-inducing properties, propanethial oxide, is released when the bulb is cut, but as it is highly water soluble, it can easily be eliminated by rinsing the peeled onion under running water.

## Leeks

With a more subtle flavor than its cousins, the leek (*Allium porrum*) is a plant originating in the Mediterranean regions, likely the Middle East. It is a vegetable with a very long history and is the source of many anecdotes, especially about its vocal properties. Aristotle, for example, was persuaded that the partridge's piercing cry was associated with a diet high in leeks. This hypothesis appealed to the Roman emperor Nero, who ate such large amounts of leek to improve the clarity of his voice that he earned the nickname of Emperor "Porophagus" (leek eater)! Last but not least, the leek is the national emblem of Wales, in honor of a memorable battle against the pagan Saxons (c. 640), during which Saint David seems to have advised King Cadwallader to distinguish between his warriors and their adversaries by having his men wear a leek in their hats. The Welsh crushed the Saxons, and this victory is celebrated every March 1, St. David's Day, by wearing a leek and eating *cawl,* a traditional dish based on leeks.

## Shallots

The Latin name for shallots (*Allium ascalonicum*) refers to the plant's place of origin, Ascalon (Ashkelon), a city in ancient Palestine on the shore of the Mediterranean Sea. Crusaders (12th century) probably introduced the shallot into Europe, where it found its natural home in France. In fact, France, including Brittany, became over time the only country producing this vegetable — hence its common name "French shallot."

Shallots look much more like garlic than onions, with a head composed of several cloves, each with a papery skin. The name shallot is often incorrectly used in North America for green onions, which are really just immature onions.

## Chives

Chives (*Allium schoenoprasum*) get their name from the Latin *cepula*, meaning "little onion." Likely native to Asia and Europe, chives were especially popular in China at least 2,000 years ago, both to flavor dishes and to treat bleeding and poisoning. On his return from his voyage to the East, Marco Polo made Europe aware of the medicinal and culinary properties of this plant.

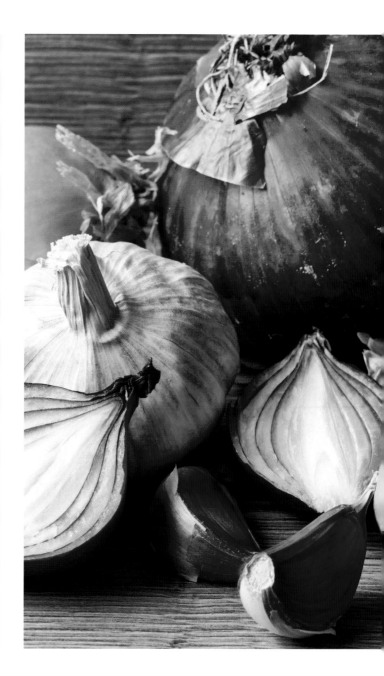

place in Egyptian customs, as indicated by the cloves discovered among the treasures in Tutankhamen's tomb (about 1300 BCE). What's more, the *Codex Ebers*, an Egyptian medical papyrus dating from this era, mentions over 20 garlic-based remedies for a variety of ailments like headache, worms, hypertension and tumors.

That said, the medicinal use of garlic was not limited to Egypt, but instead seemed to be common in most ancient civilizations. Many references to the medicinal uses of garlic were made by Aristotle, Hippocrates, Aristophanes and the Roman naturalist Pliny the Elder, with the latter going so far as to describe no fewer than 61 cures based on garlic in his *Natural History*. Garlic was recommended for treating infections, respiratory problems and digestive disorders, as well as lack of energy. Introduced into Europe by the

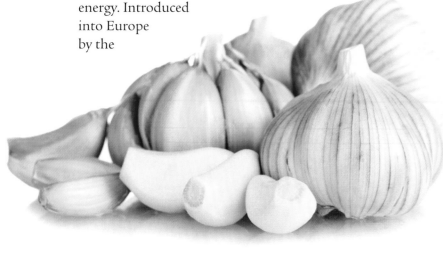

Romans, its use intensified during the Middle Ages as a way of fighting the plague and other contagious diseases, and later, in the 18th and 19th centuries, diseases like scurvy and asthma. Only in 1858 did Louis Pasteur finally confirm garlic's powerful antibacterial effects.

## The sulfur compounds in garlic and onion

Imagining the surprise of the early humans who bit into a garlic or onion bulb for the first time may make us smile, for how could they have suspected that such apparently odorless foods could release so much aroma and flavor?

This transformation is explained by the chemical changes that occur in the bulbs of members of the *Allium* family when they are broken down mechanically, somewhat as described for cruciferous vegetables. The aroma and taste so typical of the various *Allium* species are due to their high levels of several sulfur-containing phytochemicals, molecules containing an atom of sulfur in their chemical structure. Garlic can be used as a good example to illustrate the reactions that occur when cloves are crushed and added to the dish being prepared. Stored in a cool spot, the bulbs will have gradually accumulated *alliin*, garlic's main component. When the clove is crushed, the bulb's cells are broken, releasing an enzyme called *alliinase* that comes into contact with the alliin and very quickly transforms it into *allicin*, a very fragrant molecule directly responsible for the strong smell given off by the bulb just crushed. Allicin is a very plentiful (there may be as much as 5 mg/g) but highly volatile molecule; it almost instantly turns into sulfur products of varying complexity (Figure 47). Most people have heard about allicin, as all manufacturers of garlic supplements boast of the benefits of their products largely based on their allicin content. This publicity is not necessarily fraudulent, but it is nonetheless inaccurate, as these supplements do not contain allicin, but alliin; rather, it is their *potential* to cause allicin to be released that should be talked about, a potential that is directly associated with careful preservation of alliinase activity in these supplements. In addition, tests done in an independent American laboratory have shown that the amount of allicin released by these supplements ranges from 0.4 mg to 6.5 mg, depending on the manufacturer. The easiest way to know exactly how much allicin you are consuming is therefore to eat fresh garlic.

Very similar reactions occur in chopped onion; in this case, the difference in odor is mainly attributable to the slightly

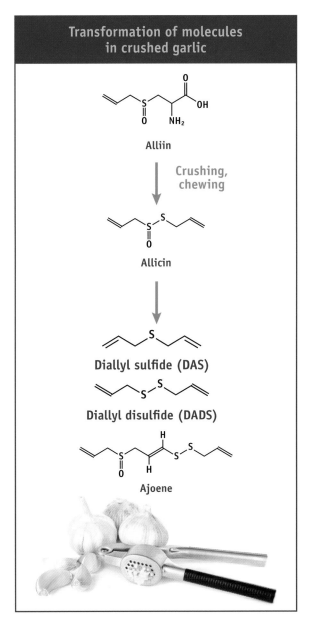

**Transformation of molecules in crushed garlic**

Alliin

Crushing, chewing

Allicin

**Diallyl sulfide (DAS)**

**Diallyl disulfide (DADS)**

**Ajoene**

**Figure 47**

different nature of the molecules found in onions, which, instead of generating allicin or its derivatives, instead produce sulfenic acids and thiosulfinates. At the same time, another enzyme (LF synthase) transforms 1-propenylsulfenic acid into a volatile and highly irritating gas called propanethial oxide. This gas spreads through the air and reaches our eyes, causing an irritation leading to tear secretion. The formation of propanethial reaches its peak 30 seconds after the onion is cut into and then decreases. With some kinds of onions this can feel like a long time!

## Garlic's anticancer properties

Currently available data on the anticancer potential of members of the garlic family suggest that they play an important role in preventing cancers of the digestive system, especially stomach, esophagus, prostate and colon cancer (Figure 48).

The first evidence of a role in preventing stomach cancer comes from epidemiological studies conducted in Yangzhong province in northeastern China, where there is a high incidence of this kind of cancer. An analysis of the dietary habits of the region's inhabitants showed that some people ate relatively little garlic and onion, and that this modest consumption was associated with a three times higher risk of getting stomach cancer. Similar results were obtained in Italy by comparing the diet of inhabitants in the north, where garlic is not much used, and those in the south, who are big garlic eaters: plentiful and frequent consumption of vegetables in the *Allium* family considerably reduces the incidence of stomach cancer.

In addition, it is thought that species in the garlic family can prevent other types of cancer, particularly prostate cancer. In a study conducted among inhabitants of the city of Shanghai, it was determined that people who ate more than 10 g per day of vegetables in the

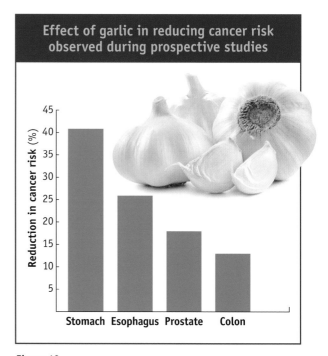

Figure 48

*Allium* family had 50 percent fewer prostate cancers than those who ate less than 2 g per day. This protective effect seems to be more pronounced for garlic than for other members of the same family. For breast cancer, on the other hand, current data do not yet allow us to say with certainty that garlic has a protective role. A Dutch study indicates that while onion consumption was associated with a major reduction in stomach cancer, it had no impact on the risk of getting breast cancer. On the other hand, French researchers have observed that the consumption of garlic and onions by women in the northeast of France (Lorraine) was associated with a decrease in breast cancer.

Currently available data show that the amounts of vegetables in the *Allium* family eaten by many Western populations are much lower than those required for a decrease in cancer risk. For example, just 15 percent of British men eat 6 g of garlic (roughly two cloves) per week, and barely 20 percent of Americans eat more than 2 g of garlic a week.

Although some researchers have theorized that allicin could be responsible for garlic's medicinal properties, its extremely high chemical volatility raises doubts as to how effectively it is absorbed by the body and its action on cells. In fact, as has already been mentioned, it is now well-known that allicin is quickly changed into a range of compounds such as ajoene, diallyl sulfide (DAS), diallyl

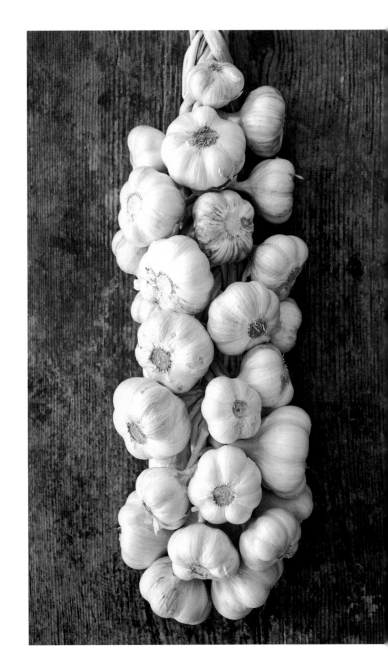

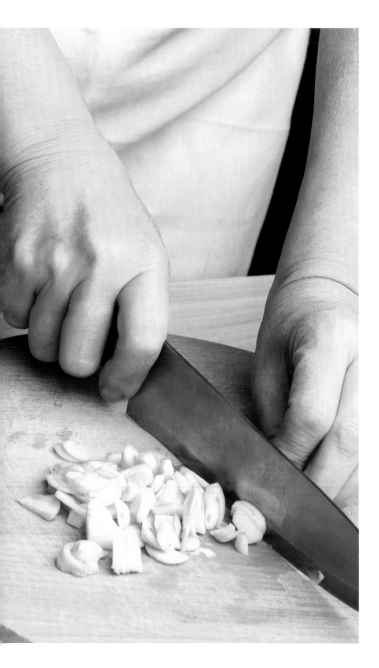

disulfide (DADS) and several other molecules, and that these derivatives have very interesting biological activities of their own. In total, at least 20 compounds derived from garlic have been studied and have shown anticancer activity. However, DAS and DADS, both oil soluble, are usually considered to be the main molecules in garlic able to play a role in cancer prevention.

In the laboratory, the anticancer properties of the compounds in garlic have mainly been studied using animal models, in which cancer onset is caused by carcinogenic chemical compounds. Generally speaking, the results obtained in animals match the observations carried out in the population: the phytochemical compounds in garlic and onions have the property of preventing the occurrence and even the progression of some cancers, especially cancers of the stomach and esophagus, although effects have also been noted for lung, breast and colon cancer. Garlic seems especially effective in preventing cancers caused by nitrosamines, a class of chemical compounds with very high carcinogenic potential. These chemical compounds are formed by the intestinal flora from nitrites, a class of food agents very frequently used as preservatives, especially in marinades and meat-based products like sausages, bacon and ham. By preventing the formation of nitrosamines, powerful carcinogens that bind with DNA, garlic's phytochemical compounds reduce the risk of these enemy compounds causing DNA mutations and, as a result, the risk of developing cancer. The protective effect of garlic with respect to nitrosamines seems to be very powerful, since DAS can even neutralize the development of lung cancer caused by NNK, an extremely toxic nitrosamine formed by the transformation of nicotine when tobacco is burned. Garlic seems to have a greater protective effect than onion, although it has been suggested that eating onions is also associated with a lower risk of developing stomach cancer.

Garlic and onion compounds might also interfere with cancer development through their effect on the systems responsible for activating and detoxifying foreign substances with carcinogenic potential (see Chapter 6). In fact, several compounds, like DAS, inhibit the enzymes that cause the activation of carcinogens, while increasing those that act to eliminate these compounds. The immediate result of these two properties is that cells are less exposed to carcinogenic agents and thus are less likely to undergo damage to their DNA, which would lead to the development of cancer. Garlic's compounds, just like those in the vegetables of the cabbage family, can as a result be considered to be first-line preventive agents, preventing cancer development at the outset.

In addition to their direct effects on carcinogenic substances, the compounds in garlic directly attack tumor cells and cause their destruction through the apoptosis process (see Chapter 2, p. 34). In fact, treating cells isolated from cancers of the colon, breast, lung and prostate, as well as from leukemias, with different garlic compounds causes significant changes in the growth of tumor cells and activates the process leading to their death. The molecule most able to cause cell death seems to be DAS, although similar effects have also been observed with other derivatives, like ajoene. Our laboratory has also observed that DAS might contribute to cancer cell death by altering their ability to express a number of proteins that allow them to resist some chemotherapy drugs.

In sum, the anticancer properties of the garlic family seem to be mainly linked to their sulfur compound content. Nonetheless, especially in the case of onions, the significant contribution of certain polyphenols must definitely not be ignored; these include quercetin, a molecule that prevents the growth of a large number of cancer cells and interferes with cancer development in animals. In any event, based on knowledge acquired to date, it is more and more certain that the compounds in garlic and onions can act as powerful inhibitors of cancer development by targeting at least two processes involved in tumor development. On the one hand, these compounds may prevent the activation of carcinogenic substances by decreasing their reactivity as well as speeding up their elimination, with both of these effects helping to reduce damage these substances cause to DNA, the main target of these carcinogens. On the other, these molecules are also able to reduce tumor propagation by interfering with the growth process of cancer cells, which causes these cells to die by apoptosis. Even though more studies are needed to identify more accurately how molecules derived from garlic and onions perform these various activities, there is no doubt at all that garlic and the other plants in this family deserve an important place in a strategy for preventing cancer through food. Garlic can frighten away much more than evil spirits and vampires!

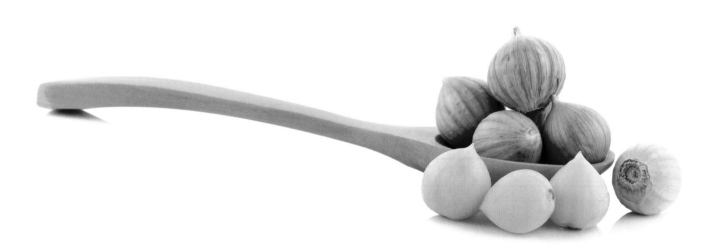

**In summary:**

- Garlic and its cousins slow down cancer development, both through their protective action against damage caused by carcinogenic substances and their ability to hinder cancer cell growth.

- The molecules responsible for these anticancer effects are released by the mechanical breakdown of these vegetables. Freshly crushed garlic is therefore by far the best source of anticancer compounds and should be chosen over supplements.

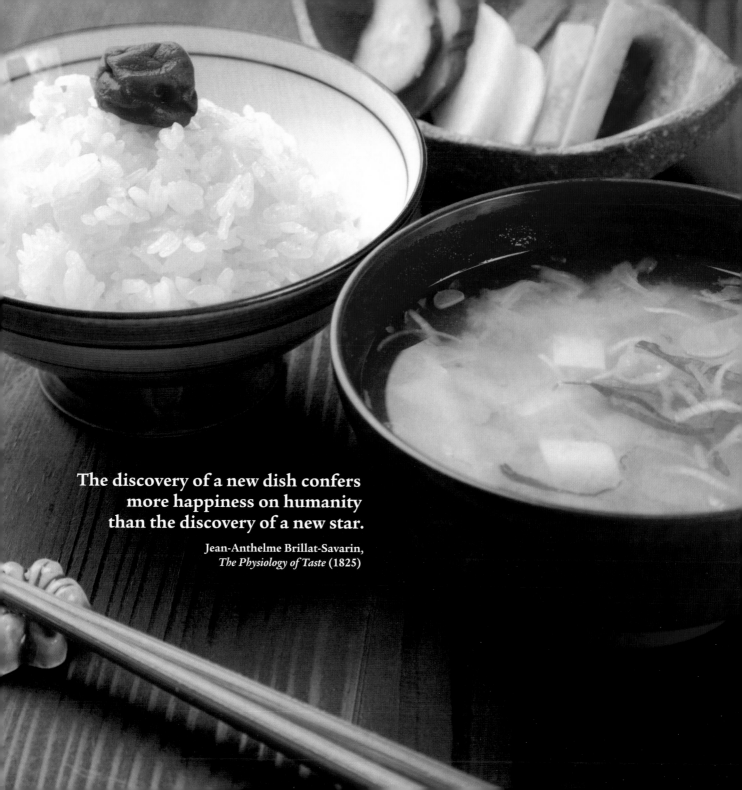

The discovery of a new dish confers
more happiness on humanity
than the discovery of a new star.

Jean-Anthelme Brillat-Savarin,
*The Physiology of Taste* (1825)

# Chapter 8

# Soy: An Incomparable Source of Anticancer Phytoestrogens

Exactly when soybean cultivation began remains unknown, but it is believed to have developed significantly about 3,000 years ago in Manchuria, in the northeast of China (now the provinces of Liaoning, Jilin and Heilongjiang), during the period corresponding to the Zhou (Tcheou) Dynasty (1122–256 BCE). At the time, soy w as considered to be one of the five sacred grains, along with barley, wheat, millet and rice, but according to some specialists this sacred character was particularly related to its use as a soil fertilizer, owing to its nitrogen-fixing properties. Indeed, soy, like the entire legume family (beans, cowpeas, peas and lentils, for example), has the ability to absorb nitrogen from the atmosphere and transfer it to the soil. These plants are therefore very profitable, as they improve the soil while creating highly nutritious substances in a relatively short time frame.

Soy seems not to have been actually included in the diet until after the discovery of fermentation techniques in the Zhou Dynasty period. In fact, the first foods made from soy were the result of fermentation, like miso and soy sauce, followed by the discovery of how to make tofu (see box, pp. 118–19). In any event, during this period, soy cultivation and fermentation methods gradually spread across southern China, reaching, in the following centuries, Korea, Japan and Southeast

*(Continued on page 120)*

# The main food sources of soy

### Fresh soybeans (edamame)

*Edamame*, a Japanese word meaning "beans on the branch," is a very popular appetizer in Japan. The pods are quickly harvested so the beans do not become too hard. After being lightly boiled, the beans are eaten directly from the pods. In the West, frozen pods are available in many supermarkets. This is definitely the tastiest and most pleasant way to eat soy, especially since the beans are also an excellent source of anticancer phytochemical compounds called isoflavones.

### Miso

Miso is a fermented paste made from a mixture of soybeans, salt and a fermenting agent (*koji*) usually derived from rice and containing the compound *Aspergillus oryzae*. The ingredients are mixed and left to ferment for a period of six months to five years. Miso appeared in Japan around 700 CE and since the Muromachi period (1338–1573) has been one of the most important ingredients in traditional Japanese cuisine. Historically, miso was used as a kind of soup to compensate for the lack of protein imposed by the Buddhist prohibition on eating meat and, even today, miso soup is the base of the traditional Japanese dish *ichiju issai* (a soup accompanied by a rice and vegetable dish). In Japan, no fewer than 10.8 pounds (4.9 kg) of miso are eaten per person per year!

### Soy sauce

Soy sauce is the main ingredient in Japanese seasoning and is undoubtedly the best known of soy-based foods in the West. This sauce is made by fermenting soybeans with a microscopic mold, *Aspergillus sojae*. Varieties of soy sauce include *shoyu*, a mixture of soybeans and wheat, *tamari*, made from soybeans only, and *teriyaki* sauce, which includes other ingredients like sugar and vinegar.

### Roasted soybeans

The beans are soaked in water and then roasted until they turn brownish. Like peanuts in appearance and taste, they are an interesting dish because of their high protein and isoflavone content. In Japan, roasted soybeans are customarily eaten on February 3 each year, at *Setsubun*, the festival celebrating the passage from winter into spring, which is where they get their name *Setsubun no mame*. In every household, during *Setsubun*, someone puts on a devil's mask and the children in the household chase him away throwing soybeans and saying, "*Fuku wa uchi, oni wa soto*" ("Happiness inside the home, the devil outside"). According to custom you have to eat the number of beans corresponding to your age to keep illness away during the year to come.

## Tofu

The production of tofu likely goes back to the Western Han period (220–22 BCE) in China. This technique relies on the pressurization of soybeans previously soaked in water, resulting in the extraction of a whitish liquid, the "milk."

Tofu is traditionally obtained by coagulating this "milk" using a natural marine compound, *nigari*, magnesium chloride (extracted from *nigari*), calcium chloride (a product made from a mineral extracted from the earth), calcium sulfate (gypsum), magnesium sulfate (Epsom salts) or acids (lemon juice, vinegar). Tofu plays a central role in all Asian cuisines, with an annual per person consumption of about 9 pounds (4 kg) compared with 3.5 ounces (100 g) in the West. Although tofu has a relatively bland flavor,

it can be greatly enhanced by ingredients added to it, as it absorbs the flavor of the foods it is prepared with.

## Soy milk

Contrary to popular belief, drinking soy milk (*tonyu*) is a recent trend in Asia and, ironically, was largely popularized by Harry Miller, an American doctor and Adventist missionary who established the first soy milk production plants in China in 1936 and in Japan in 1956. In China and Korea, only 5 percent of soy intake comes from milk, and this percentage is even lower in Japan. Many people find that soy milk has an unpleasant taste caused by strong-smelling compounds produced by an enzyme called lipoxygenase, released when the beans are pressurized. As a result, it is often sold in the form of a flavored beverage containing quite large amounts of sugar, while having far fewer phytoestrogens than traditional soy-based foods.

Asia, where the populations valued the ease of growing soy, its exceptional nutritional properties and its medicinal qualities. Even now, the consumption of soy and products derived from it are an integral part of the culinary traditions of Asian countries.

While these foods are part of the daily diet for the Japanese, Chinese and Indonesians, among other groups, it must be said that soy remains relatively overlooked in the West and that only a minority of people have incorporated it into their diets. For example, the average daily consumption of soy is approximately 2.3 ounces (65 g) per person in Japan and roughly 1.4 ounces (40 g) in China, whereas in the West it does not exceed 0.04 ounces (1 g). In the West, legumes like soy are classified under "meats and alternatives" in the food pyramid, a classification that is slightly unfair given their high levels of proteins, essential fatty acids, vitamins and minerals, as well as dietary fiber. This is truly a remarkable food whose potential still remains largely untapped in our societies — all the more so, as we will see in this chapter, given that soybeans are not only a significant source of nutrients, but are also an extremely important source of anticancer phytochemical molecules.

## Isoflavones, a key component of soy's healthful properties

The main phytochemical compounds in soy are a group of polyphenols called isoflavones. Although isoflavones are also found in other plants like chickpeas, only soy provides the body with appreciable amounts.

As Figure 49 shows, most of the products derived from soy contain a large amount of isoflavones, except for soy sauce, in which most of the molecules are broken down

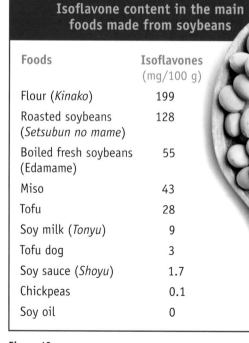

| Isoflavone content in the main foods made from soybeans | |
|---|---|
| **Foods** | **Isoflavones** (mg/100 g) |
| Flour (*Kinako*) | 199 |
| Roasted soybeans (*Setsubun no mame*) | 128 |
| Boiled fresh soybeans (*Edamame*) | 55 |
| Miso | 43 |
| Tofu | 28 |
| Soy milk (*Tonyu*) | 9 |
| Tofu dog | 3 |
| Soy sauce (*Shoyu*) | 1.7 |
| Chickpeas | 0.1 |
| Soy oil | 0 |

**Figure 49**

Source: USDA Database for Isoflavone Content of Selected Foods, 2001.

during the lengthy fermentation process, and soy oil (often sold as "vegetable oil" in supermarkets), which has none at all. The highest concentrations of isoflavones occur in soy flour (*kinako*), fresh or roasted soybeans and in some fermented products like miso. Tofu also contains a very significant amount of isoflavones.

While the consumption of soy-based foods is very low in the West, most of us nonetheless eat a lot of soy protein without being aware of it. In the West, soy-based products are referred to as "second generation" – industrial products in which animal proteins are replaced or enhanced by adding proteins derived from soy. So, rather than being considered foods in their own right as in the East, soy proteins are instead used as minor ingredients in products as varied as hamburgers, sausages, dairy products, breads, pastries and cookies.

These typically Western products contain only very few isoflavones, since they are made with protein concentrates derived from the industrial processing of soybeans (extracted using solvents derived from petroleum, processed at high temperatures and washed with alcohol-based solutions). The soy proteins obtained using these methods thus bear very little resemblance to those in the original beans. As a result, while replacing animal proteins with vegetable proteins in

these foods may offer a nutritional advantage (although the increasing use of genetically modified soy also poses significant ethical and ecological problems), adding these substitutes does not increase their isoflavone content; since the proteins used have been subjected to such processes before being incorporated into the food, the anticancer properties of soy have long disappeared.

The isoflavone content of foods derived from soy is important, as these molecules can have an influence on several events associated with the uncontrolled growth of cancer cells. The main isoflavones in soy are genistein and daidzein, with glycitein occurring in smaller amounts. An interesting characteristic of

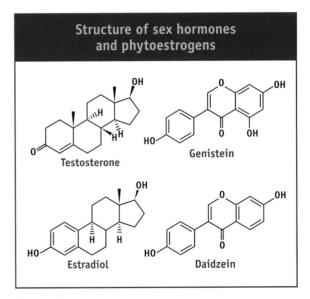

**Figure 50**

# Isoflavones, and breast and prostate cancers

Breast and prostate cancers are what are commonly known as "hormone-dependent"; that is, their growth largely depends on sex hormone levels in the blood. Under normal conditions, the amount of these hormones in the body is closely monitored by several control systems that make sure their level does not exceed a given limit. These checks are important, since some hormones, like estrogens, are powerful tissue growth stimulators, and too high a level of these hormones in the blood can cause uncontrolled growth and cancer. This is why, in the case of breast cancer, for example, people with this cancer are commonly observed to have higher blood levels of estrogens than those who are cancer free. The factors responsible for the higher levels of sex hormones in patients with these types of cancer are still very poorly understood but may include dietary elements. For example, massive intake of animal fats and the ensuing physical overload are a significant risk factor in the development of some hormone-dependent cancers like those of the endometrium and breast. Obese women have high blood levels of insulin, which, by means of very complex mechanisms, completely changes the estrogen and progesterone levels in their bodies. Suffice it to say that estrogen levels increase significantly, resulting in the overstimulation of endometrial or breast cells and excessive growth of these tissues.

In the case of prostate cancer, the contribution of androgens to the development of this disease is no longer in doubt. Excessive prostate growth seems to be inevitable, since roughly 40 percent of men aged 50 have latent prostate cancer. Several diet-based factors encourage the progression of prostate cancer, including animal fats and obesity, and controlling the growth of these latent tumors by compounds derived from foods like soy, thus takes on special importance. On the other hand, the protection soy offers against prostate cancer does not appear to be limited to its effect on androgen receptors, but also involves its inhibiting activity on growth factor receptors and angiogenesis.

isoflavones is their striking resemblance to a class of female sex hormones called estrogens, and, for this reason, these molecules are often called phytoestrogens (Figure 50). Most scientists interested in the anticancer potential of soy isoflavones consider genistein to be the main molecule responsible for these effects, owing to its ability to block the activity of several enzymes involved in the uncontrolled proliferation of tumor cells, thus bringing their growth to a halt.

As we have already mentioned, in addition to their effects on the activity of several proteins involved in the growth of tumor cells in breast or prostate cancers, phytoestrogens might also act as antiestrogens and thus decrease cells' response to these hormones. The principle is this: genistein can bind itself to the estrogen receptor, but this affinity is weaker and does not result in a response as strong as that caused by the hormone. However, genistein's structural similarity means it can occupy the space used by estrogen, thus weakening estrogen's bond with the receptor and, as a result, the biological effects ensuing from this interaction (see p. 61). This mechanism is analogous to that of tamoxifen, currently used to treat breast cancer, which has an affinity with the estrogen receptor identical to that of genistein. This property of genistein and other isoflavones to act on

hormone receptors is generating a great deal of hope for preventing hormone-dependent cancers (see box).

## Soy's anticancer properties

Hormone-dependent cancers, like breast and prostate cancer, are the main causes of death from cancer in Western countries, whereas these cancers are much rarer in Asian countries. The omnipresence of soy in the Asian diet and its almost total absence in that of Western countries suggests that the enormous differences observed in cancer rates between East and West might be linked to the ability of isoflavones like genistein to reduce the response to hormones and thus their ability to stimulate cell growth in the target tissues too dramatically.

## Isoflavones and breast cancer

A relationship between the incidence of breast cancer and soy consumption was first suggested following a study conducted in Singapore, where premenopausal women eating the most soy (2 ounces/55 g per day or more) had half as much risk of developing breast cancer as those who ate less than 0.7 ounces (20 g) daily. Other data subsequently obtained among Asian populations seem to confirm soy's protective role; for example, a major 10-year study of 21,852 Japanese women showed that daily consumption of miso soup and an isoflavone intake of 25 mg a day were associated with a stark decrease in the risk of developing breast cancer. However, the results of studies done among Western populations are less conclusive. For example, a major Californian study of 111,526 female teachers showed no correlation between soy intake and the risk of developing breast cancer; these results were also obtained in three other smaller-scale studies.

How can these differences be explained? First of all, it is important to note that in several studies where soy consumption is not associated with decreased risk the isoflavone intake is extremely low. For example, in a study done in San Francisco of non-Asian women, soy intake was only 3 mg of isoflavones per day among those who consumed the most, and

this intake was mainly linked to isoflavones derived from soy protein added to processed products. Barely 10 percent of these people ate miso or tofu more than once a month, compared with three times a day for the Japanese women at low risk of getting this disease! In fact, the isoflavone content of the group with the highest soy intake in the Californian study (3 mg/day) was half that of the group with the lowest level in the Japanese study mentioned above, in which no protective effect from soy was observed. It is therefore likely that a certain threshold of soy consumption is necessary to cause a decline in breast cancer risk, since, in all the studies that suggest this kind of protective role, eating enough soy to generate more than 25 mg of isoflavones is associated with a notable drop in breast cancer risk. Secondly, it appears that a key factor that can influence the decrease in breast cancer rates is the age at which dietary intake of products containing soy begins. In fact, when studies look at the risk of developing breast cancer by examining women's soy consumption during prepuberty and adolescence, there is a very strong relationship between soy intake in childhood and a decrease in the number of breast cancers. This early consumption of soy seems to be very important, since the breast cancer protection it provides continues to be seen later in life, even in women whose soy consumption decreases in adulthood. For example, while for female Japanese immigrants to the United States the risk of getting breast cancer is about the same as for American-born women, it has been clearly shown that this risk is much lower when these women emigrate later in life. In other words, the longer these women have been in contact with a kind of diet where soy plays a large role, the lower their risk of developing breast cancer will be later on, even if their food habits change during adulthood. These observations are consistent with certain laboratory results showing that rats fed a diet high in soy before puberty become more resistant to a carcinogenic compound causing the formation of mammary tumors than rats that were only fed soy in adulthood. Consuming soy from an early age, and especially during puberty, might therefore prove crucial to the anticancer effect of this food.

## Isoflavones and prostate cancer

As we saw in the introduction, there is no doubt that the composition of the diet plays a key role in the alarming number of prostate cancers in Western populations. As with breast cancer, Asian men have levels of this cancer several times lower than Western men, despite a similar proportion of latent tumors, which again suggests that the Eastern diet contains elements preventing the progression of these latent tumors to more serious clinical stages that can result in death.

In contrast to breast cancer, however, relatively few studies have looked at the role of soy isoflavones in the prevention of prostate cancer. One study of 8,000 men of Japanese origin living in Hawaii suggested that eating rice and tofu was associated with a decrease in the risk of developing prostate cancer. Similarly, a study of 12,395 Californian Adventists indicates that the daily consumption of at least one serving of soy results in a notable reduction (70 percent) of the risk of getting this cancer. It is therefore likely that a diet in which soy figures prominently may play an important role in preventing this disease, a hypothesis strongly supported by studies on animals.

Overall, studies conducted to date demonstrate quite clearly soy's important role in preventing breast and prostate cancers, as well as a possible reduction in risk for cancers of the uterus and lung (Figure 51). These protective effects thus show the extent to which including soy in food habits, especially during childhood and adolescence, can have extraordinary repercussions for cancer risk. Consuming foods derived from soy moderately but consistently over a long period reduces the likelihood of uncontrolled growth in breast and prostate tissues, perfectly illustrating how an active phytochemical compound can succeed in maintaining in a latent stage tumors that never stop trying to develop throughout our lives.

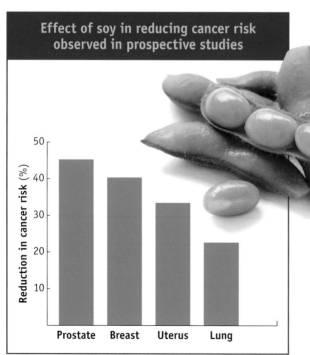

Figure 51

## The false controversy around soy

While the vast majority of researchers, doctors and nutritionists agree in saying that introducing soy into the diet is positive for health, there is nonetheless some controversy around its consumption in two very specific cases: menopausal women and women who have had breast cancer. This controversy is based on the mildly estrogenic nature of isoflavones, as well as on contradictory results obtained in laboratory animals who have undergone mammary tumor grafts. Despite all of the contradictory data reported on this subject in recent years, results recently obtained clearly show that this controversy is baseless and that eating soy is completely safe.

*Soy and menopause*
Menopause is caused by the dramatic drop in the blood levels of the female sex hormones, estrogens and progesterone, causing a halt in reproductive functions with aging. This completely normal process is often accompanied by annoying symptoms — like hot flashes and dryness of the vaginal lining — and, more importantly, by an increase in the risk of heart disease and a thinning of bone mass (osteoporosis). However, the extent

and incidence of the troublesome effects of menopause are much less significant in Asian women than in Western women: barely 14 percent of Chinese women and 25 percent of Japanese women report episodes of hot flashes, whereas 70 percent to 80 percent of Western women have to deal with these annoyances (Figure 52).

As with breast cancer, the pronounced difference in soy consumption by women in these two cultures has once again been looked at as a factor responsible for the variations observed, thus resulting in the inevitable appearance on the market of products enriched with isoflavones from soy extracts

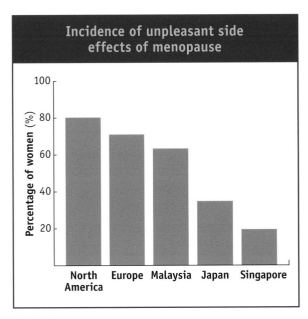

Figure 52

or red clover (another abundant source of isoflavones). These products cause a degree of concern, as formulations high in isoflavones have accelerated the development of breast cancers in laboratory mice with low estrogen levels, like those of menopausal women, which naturally brings to mind the results of the study mentioned above. These products are all the more worrisome in light of another study showing that administering a mixture of soy proteins to women aged 30 to 58 caused an increase in several blood markers associated with the risk of developing breast cancer, including, among others, the appearance of hyperplasic cells and an increase in blood estrogen levels. Overall, this data has led many people to suggest that menopausal women as well as those who have had breast cancer should refrain from eating soy.

In the specific case of menopause, the controversy is absurd and has no basis in reality; there is no doubt that soy is not harmful to women's health, whether they are pre- or postmenopausal, as attested to by the low cancer rates in countries where this food is consumed. The harmful effect in question here is actually that of *formulations enriched with isoflavones*, which have very little to do with whole soy-based foods.

Instead of gradually introducing soy into the daily diet to reach the amounts of isoflavones on a par with those consumed

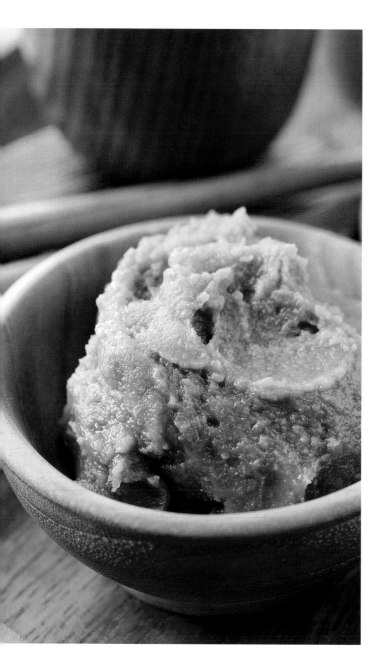

by Asians, our reflex in Western societies is to immediately isolate the active compounds in a food and market them as supplements, ideally with the highest possible amount of isoflavones to boost sales. This is the heart of the current issue concerning the "dangers" of phytoestrogens during menopause: there are Westerners who now consume enormous quantities of these molecules, disproportionate with those found in the traditional diets of Asian countries. We must remember that Asians generally consume from 1.4 ounces to 2.1 ounces (40 g to 60 g) of whole soy per day, for a maximum of 2.1 ounces (60 g) of isoflavones. In the study on the impact of miso soup on breast cancer risk, women with a low risk of getting the disease had a daily intake of 25 mg of isoflavones, whereas, in comparison, some supplements currently sold over the counter with no regulation by government bodies may contain up to 100 mg per tablet! The consequences of taking such high doses of pure isoflavones, which, like any other hormone, can cause target tissues to respond too strongly when its levels are too high, cannot be foreseen.

### Soy and breast cancer

The main aspect of the controversy around soy concerns women with breast cancer or who have battled cancer and are now in remission. More than 75 percent of breast cancers are diagnosed in women over 50 and, in the vast majority of cases, these cancers are estrogen-dependent. Since the estrogen-progesterone combination increases breast cancer risk, some researchers have put forward the hypothesis that the ability of soy isoflavones to interact with estrogen receptors might encourage the development of breast tumors in women with low estrogen levels and residual or existing tumors. The hypothesis is strengthened by the observation of the fact that administering formulations enriched with isoflavones to mice with mammary tumors, whose growth depends on estrogens, caused increased growth of these tumors.

Obviously, a large part of this controversy stems once again from the use of sources enriched with isoflavones, and in light of what we have just described for menopause, it is clear that women with breast cancer must absolutely avoid all supplements based on phytochemical compounds. Furthermore, one study showed that while sources of purified isoflavones caused an increase in the growth of mammary tumors already present in a laboratory animal, the whole food containing an equivalent amount of isoflavones had no effect whatsoever on this growth. The harmlessness of dietary soy for people with breast cancer is also suggested by epidemiological studies showing that Asian women are not only less affected by this cancer, but that those who get this

disease in spite of everything also have higher survival rates.

Many studies done in recent years clearly demonstrate that the regular consumption of soy by breast cancer survivors is completely safe and is actually associated with a significant decrease in the risk of recurrence and mortality linked to this disease. For example, a study of 10,000 women with breast cancer established that survivors who regularly consumed soy (more than 10 mg of isoflavones a day) had a 25 percent lower risk of having their cancer recur. It is also important to note that, despite the similarity of isoflavones to estrogens, studies indicate that soy in no way interferes with the effectiveness of tamoxifen or anastrozole, two drugs frequently used to treat hormone-dependent cancers. For people who have had breast cancer, there is therefore no downside to incorporating soy into food habits.

We have to keep in mind that the best study on the benefits of soy has been carried out by Asians themselves over the past several thousand years, with impressive results. Consuming soy during childhood and adolescence or during menopause has never posed any risk for these people; quite the opposite. As a result, moderate soy consumption (roughly 1.8 ounces/50 g to 3.5 ounces/100 g a day), so as to absorb about 25 to 40 mg of isoflavones daily, can have only positive effects on health by considerably reducing the risk of breast and prostate cancer, which, remember, are the main cancers affecting people in Western societies. Furthermore, the main active element in these foods, genistein, is not only a phytoestrogen but also a molecule with the power to thwart the appearance of several tumors, notably by blocking the formation of new blood vessels.

## Lignans, anticancer phytoestrogens

Although soy isoflavones are definitely the phytoestrogens that have received the most attention from the scientific and medical communities to date, there are other classes of natural phytoestrogens that can also contribute to preventing breast cancer (Figure 53). This is notably the case for lignans.

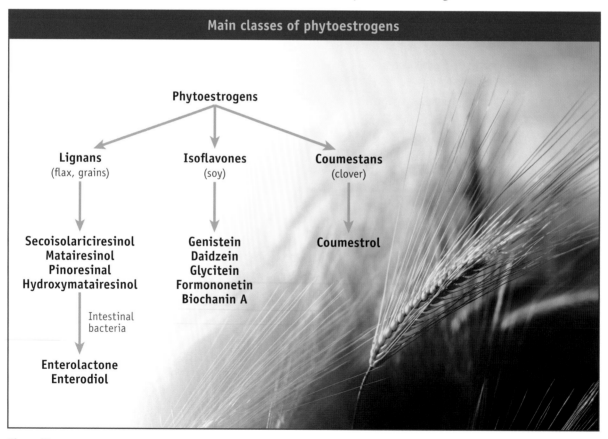

**Main classes of phytoestrogens**

Phytoestrogens

Lignans
(flax, grains)

Isoflavones
(soy)

Coumestans
(clover)

Secoisolariciresinol
Matairesinol
Pinoresinal
Hydroxymatairesinol

Genistein
Daidzein
Glycitein
Formononetin
Biochanin A

Coumestrol

Intestinal
bacteria

Enterolactone
Enterodiol

**Figure 53**

Lignans are complex compounds occurring in many plants, with flaxseeds (also called linseeds) being by far the best food source of these molecules (Figure 54). In fact, these seeds contain very high levels of *secoisolariciresinol* and its close relative *matairesinol*. These compounds are important for preventing cancers whose growth depends on estrogens, as intestinal bacteria can change them into enterolactone and enterodiol, two molecules that interfere with the bonding of estrogens to breast cells (Figure 55).

Several epidemiological studies concerning a possible role for lignans in breast cancer prevention have produced

| Secoisolariciresinol (SEC) and matairesinol (MAT) contained in foods high in lignans | | |
|---|---|---|
| Food | SEC | MAT |
| | (µg/100 g) | |
| Flaxseeds | 369,900 | 1,087 |
| Sunflower seeds | 610 | 0 |
| Peanuts | 298 | – |
| Soybeans | 273 | – |
| Cashews | 257 | 4 |
| Walnuts | 163 | 5 |
| Red beans | 153 | – |
| Rye bread | 47 | 65 |

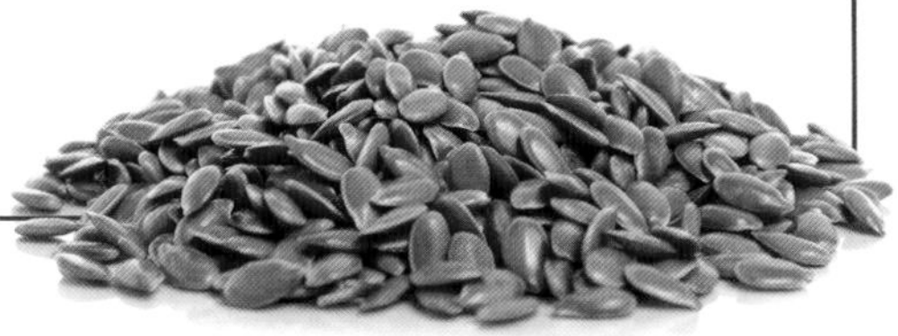

Figure 54

Structure of lignans

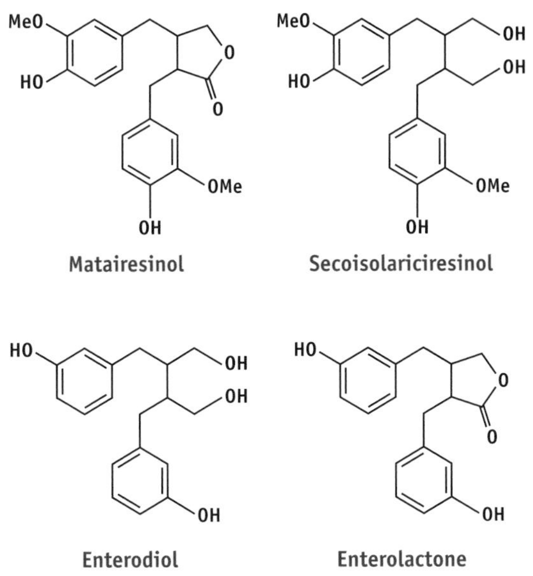

Matairesinol

Secoisolariciresinol

Enterodiol

Enterolactone

Figure 55

131

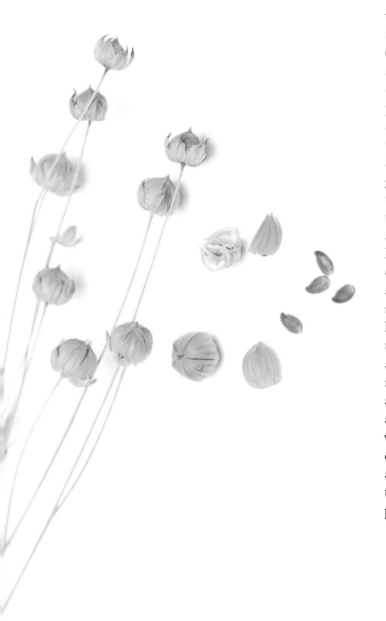

very encouraging results. In most cases, an increase in blood levels of enterolactone (produced by the transformation of secoisolariciresinol) is associated with a decreased risk of breast cancer, especially in premenopausal women, whose estrogen levels are higher. These results correspond with those of several research studies on laboratory animals who had been given mammary tumor grafts. It was observed that adding lignans to the diet prevented the development of the tumors implanted in these animals. It is also interesting to note that these studies have shown that substantial consumption of foods high in lignans is associated with a very significant reduction (70 percent) in mortality in menopausal women who have had breast cancer. Just like soy, flaxseeds are therefore a major source of phytoestrogens able to prevent both the development and recurrence of breast cancer. Since these seeds are also an outstanding source of linolenic acid, an omega-3 fatty acid able to interfere with the development of cancer by reducing chronic inflammation (see Chapter 12), they are clearly a multipurpose anticancer food that deserves a key place in any strategy for preventing cancer through diet.

**In summary:**

- The major differences in the incidence of hormone-dependent cancers (breast and prostate) between East and West could in part be attributable to the consumption of soy-based foods, especially if this consumption begins before puberty.

- The key to getting the most from soy's anticancer effects remains the consumption of whole foods, like fresh soybeans (edamame) or tofu, with the aim of getting about 1.7 ounces (50 g) per day. Isoflavone supplements, however, must be avoided.

- In addition to soy, flaxseeds are a simple and economical way to increase phytoestrogen intake. They must, however, be ground for the lignans to be changed into active phytoestrogens.

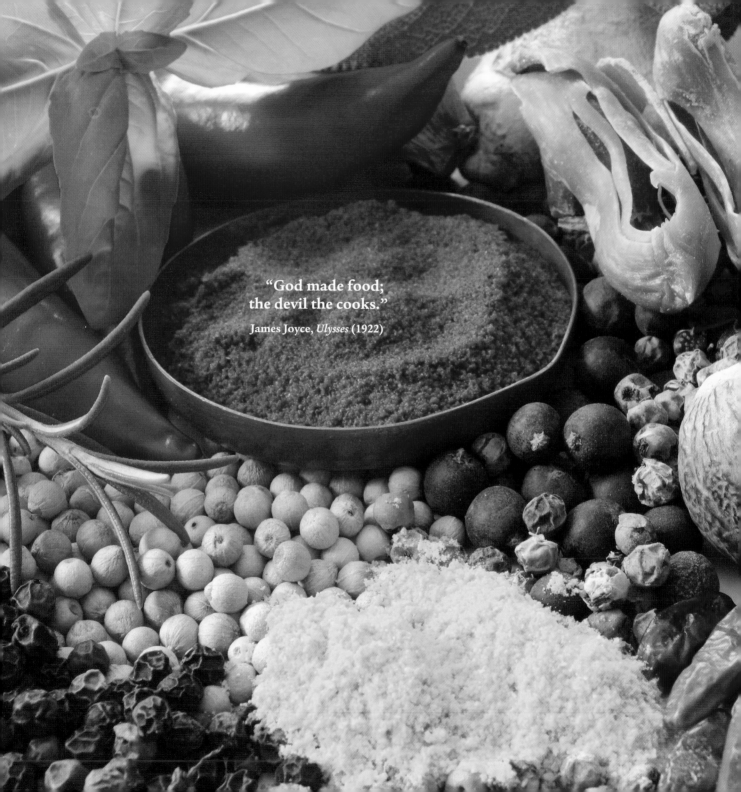

"God made food;
the devil the cooks."

James Joyce, *Ulysses* (1922)

# Chapter 9

# Spices and Herbs: A Tasty Way to Prevent Cancer

It is hard to imagine that spices could at one time have been a commodity as precious as gold and oil, so widespread have these ingredients become in today's culinary world. Yet for more than 2,000 years, the discovery of new sources of spices inflamed Europe, stirring up the greed of kings and serving as motivation for the most dangerous journeys to discover new routes leading to these riches. Without this desire for power, Vasco da Gama would not have sailed around the Cape of Good Hope, nor would Christopher Columbus or Jacques Cartier have reached and explored the Americas.

The reasons why humans attached so much importance to spices remain unclear. For some, it is likely that they were above all used to mask the bland or unpleasant taste of foods, meat especially, that had been preserved with large amounts of salt. For others, spices were a luxury commodity reserved for the wealthy that allowed them to flaunt their fortune and social status. But whether it was saffron sprinkled on Nero's path as he entered Rome or the pepper, ginger, cardamom or sugar used to pay lawyers for their work, spices were definitely a symbol of wealth and power (see box).

The word *spice* comes from the classical Latin species, meaning "kind" or "sort," and in later Latin, "spices, goods, wares." In the Middle Ages, spices were sold in specialized shops, and it was common to pay lawyers or debts in pounds of pepper or other spices.

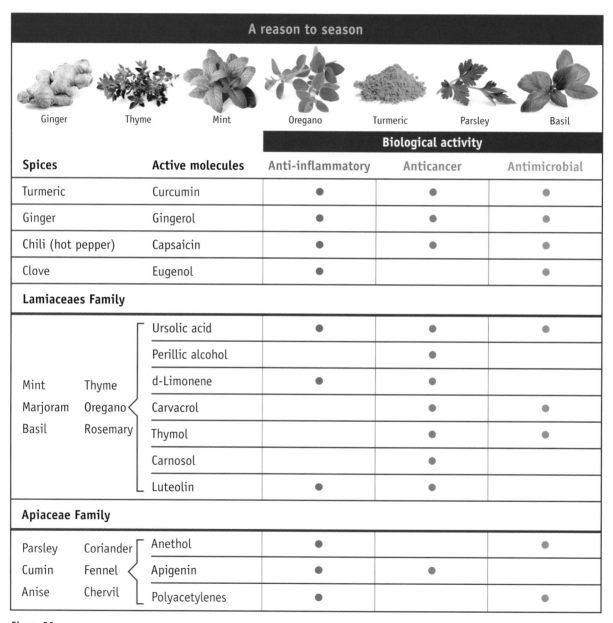

| A reason to season | | | | |
|---|---|---|---|---|

| | | **Biological activity** | | |
|---|---|---|---|---|
| **Spices** | **Active molecules** | **Anti-inflammatory** | **Anticancer** | **Antimicrobial** |
| Turmeric | Curcumin | ● | ● | ● |
| Ginger | Gingerol | ● | ● | ● |
| Chili (hot pepper) | Capsaicin | ● | ● | ● |
| Clove | Eugenol | ● | | ● |
| **Lamiaceaes Family** | | | | |
| Mint · Thyme · Marjoram · Oregano · Basil · Rosemary | Ursolic acid | ● | ● | ● |
| | Perillic alcohol | | ● | |
| | d-Limonene | ● | ● | |
| | Carvacrol | | ● | ● |
| | Thymol | | ● | ● |
| | Carnosol | | ● | |
| | Luteolin | ● | ● | |
| **Apiaceae Family** | | | | |
| Parsley · Coriander · Cumin · Fennel · Anise · Chervil | Anethol | ● | | ● |
| | Apigenin | ● | ● | |
| | Polyacetylenes | ● | | ● |

Figure 56

Since for something to be precious it must also be rare, it is also probable that spices' faraway origins played a large role in making them so mythical and sought after. In fact, setting off to discover spices meant undertaking a journey to the East, especially China and India, for, oddly, the vast majority of spices, like ginger, cardamom or saffron, come from plants that only grow in that part of the world. Given the large amounts of anticancer compounds they contain, we can only be glad to have gained access to this wealth.

## Anticancer spices

In addition to being incomparable sources of flavors and aromas, without which food would be very bland, spices and herbs commonly used in modern cooking contain molecules that can influence the processes associated with cancer development (Figure 56). In particular, one of their remarkable characteristics is their high content of anti-inflammatory molecules able to reduce inflammation of the cell environment in which precancerous tumors are found, and thus, as was explained earlier, prevent microtumors from benefiting from a climate conducive to their progression. Procarcinogenic cells have no love for well-seasoned cooking!

## Turmeric, a spice worth its weight in gold!

No spice is as closely associated with cancer prevention as turmeric. Obtained by grinding the dried rhizome of the *Curcuma longa* plant, a tropical perennial in the ginger family (the Zingiberaceae) found mainly in India and Indonesia, turmeric is a brilliant yellow spice that has always held an important place in the social, culinary and medicinal traditions of these countries. In fact, no other food discussed in this book is as specifically associated with the culture of a single country and, even now, turmeric is part of the daily diet of Indians, who consume on average from 1.5 g to 2 g per day.

In contrast, although it was already known quite long ago in Europe, turmeric has never really become part of Western culinary and medicinal traditions. It was especially valued for its color, both by the Greeks, who used it to dye their clothing, and by the dyers of the Middle Ages, who used it to obtain a very beautiful green by mixing it with indigo. Even today, turmeric remains a rather little-known spice in North America, except under the not very evocative name "E100," a widespread food coloring used in dairy products, beverages, confectionery and in some North American prepared mustards. The turmeric content of mustard may reach 50 mg/100 g; this means it would take the equivalent of 9 pounds (4 kg) of mustard per day for turmeric intake to be similar to that of Indians!

## Turmeric's therapeutic properties

Turmeric was already one of the 250 medicinal plants mentioned in a series of medical treatises dating from approximately 3000 BCE, written in cuneiform on stone tablets and compiled by King Ashurbanipal (669–627 BCE) (*The Assyrian Herbal*, so called by its discoverer, Englishman R.C. Thompson).

Interest in turmeric in the search for foods to prevent cancer actually stems mainly from the many medicinal traditions in places where this spice is widespread. Turmeric is one of the main components of traditional Indian medicine, known as ayurvedic medicine (*ayur*: life, and *vedic*: knowledge). Probably humanity's oldest medical tradition (the first school was founded around 800 BCE), Ayurvedic medicine is the cornerstone of the main schools of traditional Asian medicine (Chinese, Tibetan and Islamic) and is still practiced in India, where it is considered a viable alternative to Western medicine. In this tradition, turmeric is considered to have the property of purifying the body and is used to treat a very wide variety of physical disorders, such as digestive problems, fever, infections, arthritis and dysentery, as well as jaundice and other liver problems.

Indians are not alone in attributing health benefits to turmeric. Chinese medicine uses it mainly to treat liver disorders, congestion and bleeding. Turmeric was especially popular in the Okinawa region, located near the Ryukyu Islands, south of Japan, where it was used under the name *ucchin* throughout the Ryukyuan Kingdom period (12th to 17th centuries), both as a medicine or spice and as a coloring agent for *takuan*, a marinated radish. After the islands were invaded by the Satsuma clan in 1609, turmeric fell into disuse, but it has recently resurfaced and has once again become very popular, especially as a tea. Famous for their longevity (86 years for women and 77 for men) and their abnormally high number of centenarians (40 per 100,000 inhabitants as compared to 15 per 100,000 in the rest of Japan), the inhabitants of Okinawa consider *ucchin* to be one of the foods contributing to their exceptional health.

The French word for turmeric, "curcuma," is derived from the Arab word *kourkoum*, meaning "saffron"; in fact, turmeric is also called "saffron of the Indies." Marco Polo mentioned in his tales in 1280 the discovery of "a plant with all the properties of real saffron, the same aroma and the same color, and yet it is not saffron." Turmeric was also formerly called "terra merita," likely referring to its distant origins or its value. While "terra merita" is no longer used in French, this expression is the root of the English name *turmeric*.

Turmeric and curry must not be confused. The word "curry" comes from the Tamil *kari*, a term denoting a dish cooked in a spicy sauce. This word was misinterpreted by the British colonizers, who associated it instead with the spices used in preparing dishes. Curry powder is not therefore a spice but rather a mixture of spices, which nonetheless contains large amounts of turmeric (from 20 percent to 30 percent), usually mixed with coriander, cumin, cardamom, fenugreek and various peppers (cayenne, red and black). There are many kinds of curry and they vary in pepper content, which can sometimes cause hot flushes in unwise diners! And you won't forget the experience, if observations showing that Indians have the lowest rates of Alzheimer's disease in the world, five times lower than in Western populations, can be relied on.

## Turmeric's anticancer effects: Curcumin

There is some consensus in the scientific community to suggest that turmeric could be responsible for the huge differences in the rates of certain cancers in India and in Western countries, the United States for example (Figure 57), and might explain the dramatic increase in the incidence of cancers following the migration of Indians to Western countries (Figure 58). This hypothesis is based on the fact that turmeric is almost exclusively consumed in India, and in very large quantities, as well as on an impressive number of laboratory results on the anticancer effect of turmeric's main component, curcumin.

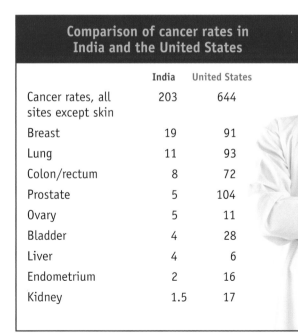

### Comparison of cancer rates in India and the United States

|  | India | United States |
|---|---|---|
| Cancer rates, all sites except skin | 203 | 644 |
| Breast | 19 | 91 |
| Lung | 11 | 93 |
| Colon/rectum | 8 | 72 |
| Prostate | 5 | 104 |
| Ovary | 5 | 11 |
| Bladder | 4 | 28 |
| Liver | 4 | 6 |
| Endometrium | 2 | 16 |
| Kidney | 1.5 | 17 |

**Figure 57**
Source: GLOBOCAN 2000, *Cancer Incidence, Mortality and Prevalence Worldwide*, 2001.

Curcuminoids are the main compounds in turmeric (approximately 5 percent of the weight of the dried root) and are responsible not only for turmeric's yellowish color, but also for the beneficial effects associated with this spice. Turmeric's main component, curcumin (Figure 59), has various pharmacological actions, including antithrombotic, hypocholesterolemic and antioxidant (several times higher than vitamin E) properties, as well as very high anticancer potential.

Curcumin's anticancer effect in laboratory animals has been well established by the

observation that administering this molecule to mice prevents the occurrence of tumors caused by various carcinogens. These studies have shown that curcumin could be useful in preventing and treating several types of cancer, including stomach, intestinal, colon, skin and liver cancer, both at the initiation and developmental stages of cancer. These results are in agreement with other studies indicating that curcumin blocks the growth of an impressive number of cells from human tumors, notably those taken from leukemias, and from colon, breast and ovarian cancers. Generally

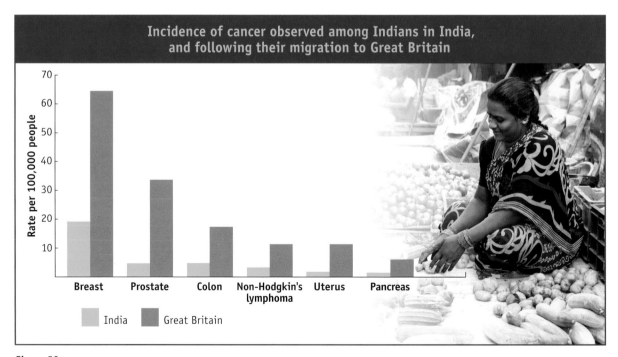

**Incidence of cancer observed among Indians in India, and following their migration to Great Britain**

Rate per 100,000 people

Breast　Prostate　Colon　Non-Hodgkin's lymphoma　Uterus　Pancreas

India　Great Britain

**Figure 58**

speaking, these effects seem to be linked to the blockage of certain processes necessary to cancer cells' survival, which renders them unable to avoid death by apoptosis. Studies also suggest that curcumin prevents the formation of new blood vessels by angiogenesis, thus depriving tumors of their energy source.

Several studies have confirmed curcumin's cancer-preventing potential by using experimental models in which cancer is not caused by carcinogenic substances but instead by factors more representative of the risks humans are exposed to. For example, in genetically modified mice that spontaneously develop polyps in the gastrointestinal tract, a significant risk factor for colon cancer, the administration of curcumin has been able to significantly slow (by 40 percent) the development of these polyps. This effect of curcumin seems mainly related to the blockage of tumors' dangerous progression stage, which suggests that adding curcumin to the diet of people in whom these polyps have already been detected might help prevent them from degenerating into a more advanced cancer.

It actually seems that colon cancer is one of the cancers curcumin could have the most impact on, as it lowers the levels of an enzyme called cyclooxygenase-2 (COX-2), responsible for producing molecules that cause inflammation (aspirin and the anti-inflammatory Celebrex are inhibitors of this enzyme). This property might have a beneficial effect on colon cancer, as studies carried out to date indicate that these anti-inflammatories reduce its incidence. Administering curcumin orally causes a dramatic reduction in the inflammatory molecules formed by COX-2 in the blood. This effect is very interesting, especially in light of the latest results showing that synthetic anti-inflammatories have side effects that can be considerable and could limit their future use in preventing colon cancer. More than 20 clinical trials are currently underway to measure the effectiveness

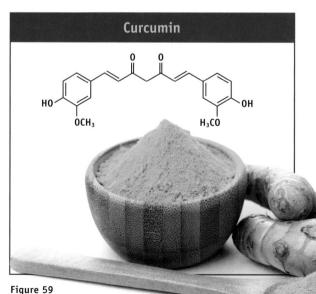

**Curcumin**

Figure 59

of turmeric and curcumin in treating various cancers (colon, breast, pancreas, melanoma). Preliminary results are encouraging, as turmeric and curcumin do not produce side effects (or very few), even in relatively high doses, and some patients respond favorably to treatment. Curcumin improves the response to chemotherapy in women with advanced forms of breast cancer. During a study carried out on patients with cancer of the pancreas in the terminal phase, administering curcumin led to a dramatic reduction (73 percent) in tumor size in a patient and stabilized the disease. These remarkable responses illustrate the powerful anticancer action of this molecule in terms of cancer prevention.

One aspect that might appear to reduce curcumin's effectiveness is its low bioavailability, that is, its low level of absorption by the body. It is important to note, however, that a molecule in pepper, piperine, increases the absorption of curcumin by more than a thousand times, a property that could no doubt be used to maximize the molecule's benefits (see Figure 97, p. 249). Greater absorption of curcumin has also been observed in the presence of ginger and cumin. Popular wisdom has perhaps once again beaten science to the punch, since pepper, ginger and cumin have always been essential elements of curry ... this increase in the bioavailability of curcumin has also been observed for other phytochemical compounds: for example, the simultaneous administration of curcumin and quercetin, a polyphenol found in many fruits and vegetables, caused a 60 percent reduction in the growth of precancerous polyps in patients at high risk of colorectal cancer owing to a genetic mutation passed on through heredity (familial rectocolic polyposis). All of these examples clearly illustrate the concept of culinary synergy, in which one food increases the impact of another eaten at the same meal.

## Anticancer herbs

Most of the herbs now used in cooking are from the Lamiaceae (mint, thyme, marjoram, oregano, basil, rosemary, etc.) and Apiaceae (parsley, coriander, cumin, chervil, fennel) families. Most of these plants come from the Mediterranean basin, where they have played a fundamental role in the development of the region's culinary traditions.

The Lamiaceae and Apiaceae all have highly fragrant leaves, owing to their high levels of essential oils containing aromatic molecules from the terpene family. Terpenes also have the important characteristic of interfering with cancer development by blocking the function of several oncogenes involved in cancer cell growth. For example, adding terpenes (carvacrol, thymol, perillic alcohol) to cancer cells taken from a wide variety of tumors considerably reduces their proliferation and, in some cases, causes their death. Adding carnosol (a terpene especially plentiful in rosemary) to the diet of mice genetically predisposed to get colon cancer prevents the development of cancer by correcting the defects in intestinal cells that cause the disease in the mice. It should also be noted that the herbs in this family contain ursolic acid, a multipurpose anticancer molecule with the ability to directly attack cancer cells, prevent angiogenesis and block COX-2 production, thus reducing inflammation.

This anticancer activity is not however limited to the terpenes in these herbs, as luteolin (Figure 60) and apigenin, two polyphenols especially plentiful in thyme, mint and parsley, also display many anticancer activities. Apegenin, for example, inhibits the growth of an impressive number of cancer cells, notably those derived from the main cancers occurring in Western countries: breast, colon, lung and prostate cancers. Although apigenin is a completely different molecule from those found in other spices and herbs, the mechanisms involved in its anticancer effects are in many ways similar; apigenin has a direct impact on both cancer cells and angiogenesis. Luteolin and apigenin prevent the PDGF growth factor from recruiting the muscle cells essential for establishing the blood vessel network tumors need to grow. This inhibiting effect is even more interesting in that it occurs in relatively weak concentrations, similar to those of Gleevac, a chemotherapy drug used in treating certain cancers (Figure 61).

It is also interesting to note that a recent study showed that women who consumed the highest amounts of apigenin had 21 percent less risk of getting ovarian cancer than those whose intake of this molecule was lower. Even though herbs are usually consumed in limited amounts and, as a

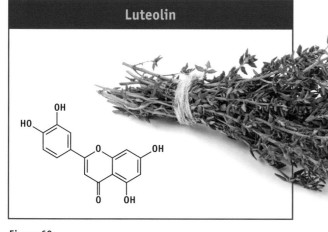

**Luteolin**

**Figure 60**

result, are not major sources of polyphenols, it is nonetheless the case that eating these herbs regularly can help prevent diseases. For example, studies have shown that people who ate large amounts of parsley had a considerable accumulation of apigenin in the bloodstream, in amounts large enough to block some of the processes involved in cancer cell growth. Furthermore, since apigenin is eliminated relatively slowly from the body, the regular consumption of foods containing large quantities of this molecule (like parsley or celery) can also contribute to achieving high enough blood levels of apigenin.

In conclusion, research done in recent years indicates that many spices and herbs used in the world's culinary traditions have anticancer properties. This effect is especially well documented for turmeric, but it is interesting to note that all spices and herbs, whether ginger, chili, clove, fennel or cinnamon, among others, also contain molecules with anti-inflammatory properties that have the potential to block the development of precancerous cells. The culinary use of spices and herbs is therefore not only essential to enhance the flavor of our daily dishes, but it must also be considered as a way of adding to the diet a concentrate of biologically active compounds with powerful anticancer action. It just goes to show that cancer prevention can also be a matter of good taste!

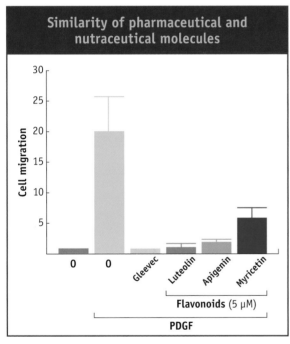

Figure 61

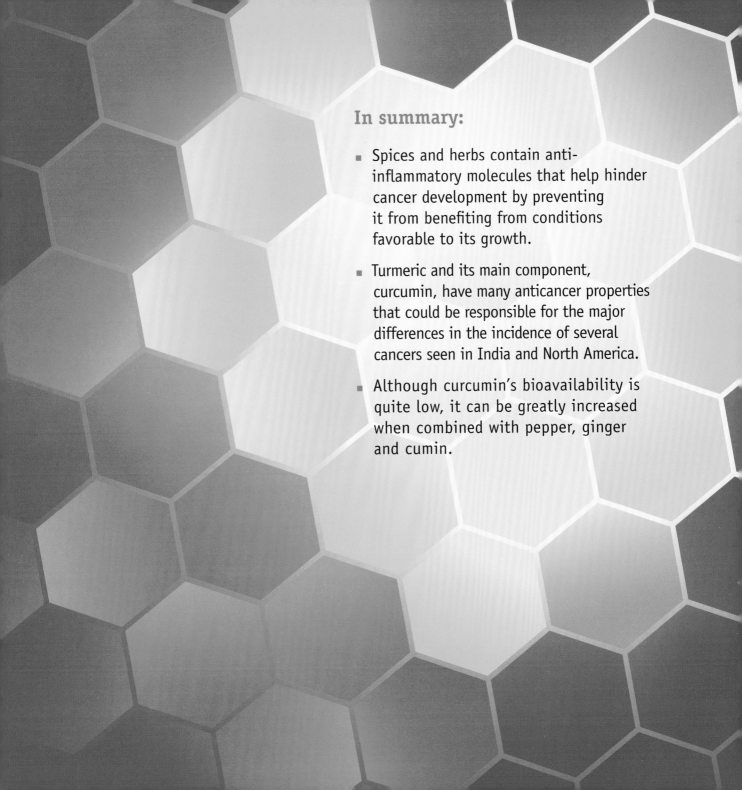

**In summary:**

- Spices and herbs contain anti-inflammatory molecules that help hinder cancer development by preventing it from benefiting from conditions favorable to its growth.

- Turmeric and its main component, curcumin, have many anticancer properties that could be responsible for the major differences in the incidence of several cancers seen in India and North America.

- Although curcumin's bioavailability is quite low, it can be greatly increased when combined with pepper, ginger and cumin.

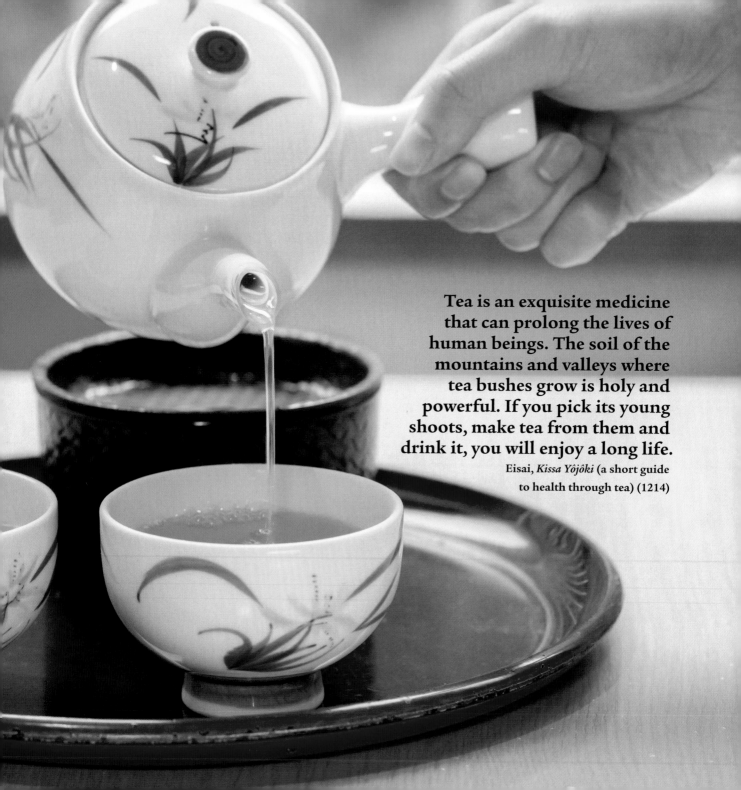

Tea is an exquisite medicine that can prolong the lives of human beings. The soil of the mountains and valleys where tea bushes grow is holy and powerful. If you pick its young shoots, make tea from them and drink it, you will enjoy a long life.

Eisai, *Kissa Yôjôki* (a short guide to health through tea) (1214)

# Chapter 10

# Green Tea: A Cancer-Fighting Balm for the Soul

It is impossible to properly approach the concept of preventing cancer through diet without paying special attention to green tea. Much more than a simple beverage, green tea has become over the centuries an essential part of the customs of Asian countries, not only from a gastronomic point of view, but also for preventing and treating diseases. Unfortunately, as with the other foods of Asian origin discussed in this book, green tea remains less well-known in the West than in the East and, according to some, this difference contributes to accentuating the gap between cancer rates among Asians and Westerners. Green tea is an outstanding source of very powerful anticancer molecules, making it one of the key elements of any diet designed

to prevent the occurrence of cancer. And, even better, the medicine tastes delicious!

The discovery of tea was likely the result of human beings' many attempts to identify plants with properties beneficial to health. According to a Chinese legend, this discovery dates back to 5,000 years BCE, when the Emperor Shen Nong, while boiling water to purify it, saw a few leaves blown by the wind fall into the simmering water. Intrigued by the color and the exquisite fragrance that arose from it, he decided to taste it and was surprised to discover a flavorful beverage with many fine qualities.

In fact, many specialists think that the discovery of tea probably took place just a few centuries before our era. The works of

# The production of tea

**Green tea.** Green teas are teas that undergo the least processing and whose production even today is still largely handcrafted. Just three stages are necessary for the production of these teas, with each being crucial to the quality of the final product. The first stage consists of briefly *steam-roasting* the freshly picked leaves; this deactivates in a few seconds the enzymes responsible for fermentation and preserves the leaves' original color. After being cooled and dried, the leaves are subjected to the second stage, *rolling*, in which they are rolled up into little balls to break down their cells and release their flavors. In the third stage, they are dried by *desiccation* by rolling them into smaller and smaller shapes until they look like needles. All of these stages, from picking the leaves to how they are processed, determine the quality of the product. For example, ordinary teas, called *sencha*, are more refreshing, whereas the shaded teas, called *gyokuru*, are milder. The first crop, in May, provides the most delicate and tender leaves, used in the production of *sencha* and *gyokuru* teas. The summer crop produces a stronger tea, *bencha*, containing less caffeine, however. *Gyokuru* teas are considered by some to be the best green teas in the world.

**Black tea.** Black tea production resembles that of green tea except that the roasting stage takes place at the end of the process rather than at the beginning. First, the leaves are wilted by exposing them to heat to decrease their water content and cause the release of the polyphenol oxidase, the enzyme responsible for the fermentation (oxidation) of the leaves. They are then rolled to break down their cells before being fermented, a reaction during which polyphenols are converted into black pigments. Finally, roasting stops the fermentation process by deactivating the enzyme, as well as eliminating excess moisture. As with green tea, the quality of black obtained is directly related to the producer's know-how. Darjeeling tea, one of the most famous black teas, is also one of the rare black teas to contain significant levels of catechins, the anticancer molecules associated with tea.

**Oolong tea.** This tea, which is consumed less widely, is called semi-fermented; that is, its production resembles that of black tea, but with a shorter fermentation stage. As a result, this tea may be considered to be an intermediary between green tea and black tea. Formosa (Taiwan) oolong, slightly blacker than China oolong, is the most sought after.

Confucius (551–479 BCE), as well as those written during the Han period (from 206 BCE–220 CE), mention it several times, but at the time its use was limited to medicinal treatments. Only later did tea gradually become part of everyday life, in particular under the Tang dynasty (618–907), when it became a daily beverage, to be enjoyed for itself as well as for its restorative properties, and growing and processing tea became a noble art, just like calligraphy, painting and poetry. Tea consumption had become so widespread by the end of the eighth century that it (obviously) became subject to a tax, the Chinese thus establishing a custom that would be copied by the British a few centuries later and have serious consequences for the stability of their empire. To bail out their treasury, the English committed the error of excessively taxing some of the commodities destined for their colonies, including tea, arousing the anger of their American colony, and resulting in 1773 in the plundering of 342 chests of tea from English ships anchored in Boston. The Boston Tea Party, as it became known, is today still considered to be the first step in the process that was to lead to the independence of the United States.

Japan contributed greatly to the boom in tea, and it is there that some of the best green teas are processed today. Although it was introduced into Japan in the eighth

century, tea growing only began to take permanent hold and gradually become an essential part of the Japanese soul in the 12th century. The importance of tea in this culture is magnificently illustrated by the *chanoyu*, a very elaborate tea ceremony based on the teaching of harmony, respect, purity and tranquillity. Although this ceremony is less common today, the soul of *chanoyu* still strongly imbues the very close relationship between the Japanese and green tea.

## The green and the black

Tea is produced from the young shoots of the *Camellia sinensis* bush, a tropical plant that likely originated in India and was brought to China via the Silk Road. In its wild state, this plant can grow as large as a tree, but under cultivation it is maintained in the form of a bush, both to make it easier to harvest and to stimulate the formation of young leaf shoots. As the box opposite indicates, the three main types of tea, whether green, black or oolong, are all obtained from the leaves of *C. sinensis* (or *C. sinensis assamica*, in India), but their characteristics vary depending on the method used to produce the dried leaves.

Tea is, after water, of course, the world's most popular beverage: 15,000 cups of tea are drunk every second on the planet, which equals

500 billion cups of tea a year, an average of 100 cups per person. Black tea is currently the most popular, with 78 percent of worldwide consumption, whereas green tea is preferred by 20 percent of tea drinkers. Black tea is especially popular in the West, where it represents roughly 95 percent of the tea consumed; conversely, it is extremely rare in Asia, which is very loyal to the original green tea. In Asia, 95 percent of black tea is consumed in India, where it is a relatively recent custom and strongly influenced by the country's British colonial past.

Despite their common origin, green and black teas have a completely different chemical composition. In fact, during the fermentation stage in the processing of black tea, dramatic changes take place in the nature of the polyphenols initially found in the tea leaves, causing them to oxidize and produce black pigments, called theaflavins. This transformation has very important consequences for cancer prevention, as the polyphenols in fresh tea leaves have anticancer properties and their oxidation eliminates nearly all of this potential. In terms of cancer prevention, green tea thus has a huge advantage over its oxidized derivative, black tea. Given the major differences in properties, it is logical to think that a simple change in tea consumption habits could have a large influence on the reduction of the number of cancers in the West. Actually, green tea was at one time a Western

custom too; the reasons that caused people to adopt black tea were mainly political and economic, and not related to any particular Western aversion to green tea.

When it was introduced into Europe in the 1600s, likely by Portuguese merchants, most tea was definitely green, since the fermentation techniques required to produce black tea (which the Chinese instead called "red tea," *hong cha*) had just begun to appear in China under the Ming Dynasty (1368–1644) and were not yet very widespread. However, the long sea voyages to the importing countries would no doubt have a negative effect on green tea's fragile taste properties (the first delivery of tea to Canada, in 1716, took more than a year to arrive at its destination), whereas black tea could easily cover long distances without any noticeable change of taste. This was bound to encourage people to drink more black tea. In spite of everything, green tea remained extremely popular in England up to the middle of the 19th century and, because of its more attractive appearance, could be sold for a higher price than black tea. However, when Chinese producers realized that the look of green tea could boost sales, they had the peculiar reaction of trying to enhance the color of the leaves by adding chemical compounds (likely copper salts) during processing. Once discovered, this obviously caused a scandal and the permanent abandonment of the consumption of green tea. It is still absent from the English market, although the British are the world's largest tea consumers. Subsequently, the English colonization of India led to the development of tea growing on a large scale in the country, which definitively established black tea as Europe's exclusive source of tea. Even today, India remains the main producer of black tea, with 38 percent of worldwide production.

Less "monoteaist" than the English, North Americans, until the early 1930s, drank as much green tea as black tea, actually showing a clear preference for green tea at one time. For example, Canadian archives indicate that in 1806, 90,000 pounds (40,800 kg) of green tea were imported into Canada, compared with just 1,500 pounds (680 kg) of black tea! It was not until the beginning of the war between China and Japan over the control of Manchuria, in 1931, that green tea exports to North America plummeted and tea consumers had to fall back on black tea.

Reconnecting with these traditions would be a good idea, as green tea is truly in a separate class in terms of its anticancer properties, and replacing black tea with green tea could have a considerable impact on cancer rates in Western countries.

## The anticancer properties of green tea

Tea is a complex beverage, made up of several hundred different molecules that give it its characteristic aroma, taste and astringency (Figure 62). A third of the weight of tea leaves contains a class of polyphenols called flavanols, or more commonly *catechins*, and these molecules are the main source of green tea's anticancer potential.

Like all of the other polyphenols, catechins are complex molecules that play an extremely important role in the plant's physiology, as they possess antifungal and antibacterial properties useful for resisting the invasion of a large number of pathogenic agents. Green tea

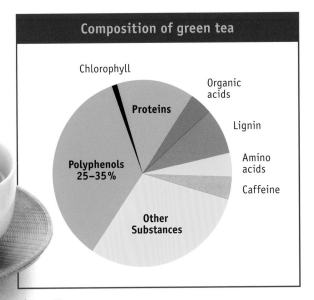

**Composition of green tea**

Chlorophyll
Organic acids
**Proteins**
Lignin
**Polyphenols 25–35%**
Amino acids
Caffeine
**Other Substances**

**Figure 62**

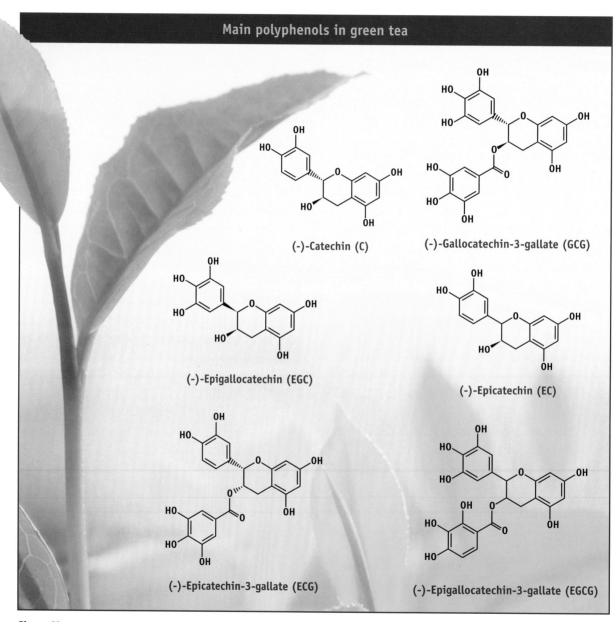

**Main polyphenols in green tea**

(-)-Catechin (C)

(-)-Gallocatechin-3-gallate (GCG)

(-)-Epigallocatechin (EGC)

(-)-Epicatechin (EC)

(-)-Epicatechin-3-gallate (ECG)

(-)-Epigallocatechin-3-gallate (EGCG)

**Figure 63**

contains several catechins, including EGCG or epigallocatechin gallate, the main catechin in green tea, with the highest anticancer potential (Figure 63).

It is important to note that the catechin profile of green tea varies greatly depending on where it is grown, the diversity of plants used, the harvesting season and the processing methods. In other words, it is not because the label on a product says it is a green tea that it necessarily contains large quantities of anticancer molecules. Analysis of several types of green tea shows that there are very significant variations in the EGCG content released by infusing the leaves (Figure 64) and that, generally speaking, Japanese green teas contain more EGCG than Chinese green teas.

We should mention as well that the length of time the leaves are steeped is also an extremely important factor in the tea's polyphenol content, and that a long infusion (from eight to 10 minutes) allows more polyphenols to be extracted. A tea of mediocre quality, steeped for a short time, may thus contain almost 60 times fewer polyphenols than a tea of excellent quality properly brewed (Figure 65). It goes without saying that these

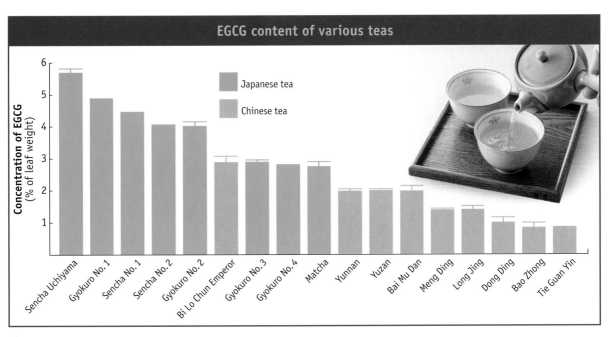

**Figure 64**

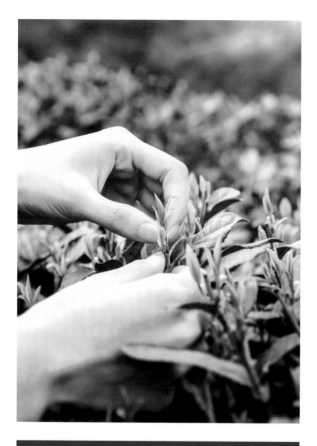

huge variations can greatly influence the potential for cancer prevention associated with green tea consumption.

The very wide variability in the composition of the green tea that individuals consume also makes it hard to analyze its cancer protection effect by means of epidemiological studies. In spite of all this, several studies done in recent years suggest that green tea has a beneficial action for cancer prevention (Figure 66), with this effect being more pronounced for mouth, colon and prostate cancers (the metastatic form of the disease). In the latter case, one study showed that regular consumption of green tea (but not black tea) resulted in an accumulation of polyphenols in prostatic tissue, a reduction in the pro-inflammatory protein NFkB and a decrease in prostate-specific antigen, a marker for this disease. A protective effect for breast, liver, bladder, lung and stomach cancer has also been suggested. These differences are likely largely connected to the extreme variations in polyphenols contained in green tea, and new studies aiming to clearly determine green tea's anticancer potential should as a result consider tea intake from the point of view of the quantity of polyphenols consumed rather than the volume of tea ingested. In this sense, it is interesting to note that the measurement of

| Variation in polyphenol content in green tea | |
|---|---|
| | mg of polyphenols in one cup |
| Tie Guan Yin tea brewed for 2 minutes | 9 |
| Gyokuru tea brewed for 10 minutes | 540 |

Figure 65

catechins and their metabolites in urine shows that people who excrete the largest amounts of these molecules (and who have therefore been more exposed to their anticancer actions) have a 60 percent lower risk of getting colon cancer.

Meanwhile, there are many good reasons to believe that drinking green tea may significantly lower the risk of developing cancer. EGCG inhibits the growth *in vitro* of several cancer cells, including cell lines of leukemia and of kidney, skin, breast, mouth and prostate cancers. These effects are important, as studies done on animals have shown that green tea prevents the development of several tumors caused by carcinogens, mainly skin, breast, lung, esophageal, stomach and colon cancers. This protective effect does not seem to be limited to tumors caused by carcinogenic substances, since the addition of green tea to the diet of genetically modified mice that spontaneously develop prostate cancer considerably reduces the growth of these tumors; this occurs with doses that can be obtained by regularly drinking green tea.

One of the aspects of green tea's protection that may contribute the most to limiting cancer development is its powerful action on the angiogenesis process. Of all the nutrition-related molecules identified to date, EGCG is the most powerful for blocking VEGF receptor activity, a key factor in the triggering of angiogenesis. What is most interesting is that this receptor inhibition is very fast and only requires weak concentrations of the molecule, easily attainable by drinking a few cups of green tea daily. Angiogenesis inhibition is definitely one of the main mechanisms by which green tea can help prevent cancer.

We cannot rewrite history, but given all of the anticancer properties associated with green tea, we cannot help but

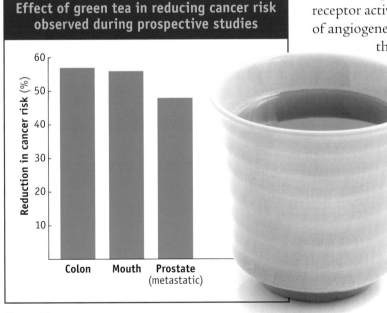

**Effect of green tea in reducing cancer risk observed during prospective studies**

Reduction in cancer risk (%)

Colon    Mouth    Prostate (metastatic)

**Figure 66**

think that cancer would perhaps be a lighter burden in our societies if Westerners had retained their taste for green tea, instead of replacing it with black tea. The situation, however, is far from being irreversible, and tea lovers curious to explore the possibility of changing their habits will be pleasantly surprised by green tea's attractive appearance, refreshing taste and four times lower caffeine content. More than just part of a diet for preventing cancer, green tea can become the "soul" of this diet, a symbol of the ease and pleasure of providing the body with a daily dose of anticancer molecules, in a relaxed and uncomplicated way. Tea master Sen no Rikyu (1522–1591) said that the tea ritual was nothing more than boiling water, preparing tea and drinking it. In light of what we have learned since then, we might add preventing cancer to this list.

**In summary:**

- Contrary to black tea, green tea contains large amounts of catechins, molecules with a host of anticancer properties.

- To maximize the protection tea offers, it is preferable to choose Japanese green teas, richer in anticancer molecules, and let the tea brew for eight to 10 minutes to extract the most molecules possible.

- Always drink freshly brewed tea (avoid thermoses) and space your drinking out throughout the day.

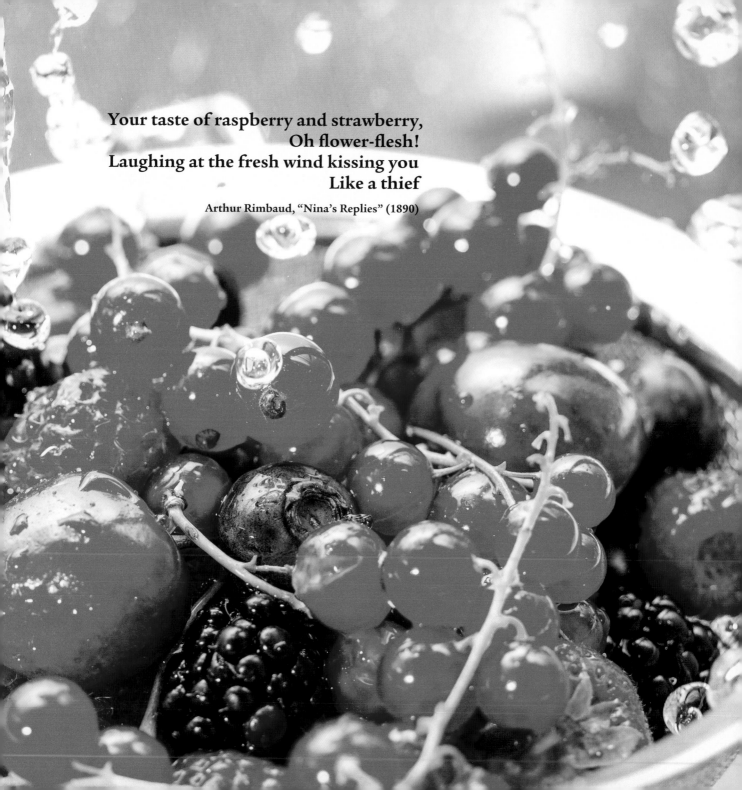

Your taste of raspberry and strawberry,
Oh flower-flesh!
Laughing at the fresh wind kissing you
Like a thief

Arthur Rimbaud, "Nina's Replies" (1890)

# Chapter 11

# A Passion for Berries

Synonymous with lightness and freshness, and sources of the most delicate scents, the most intense colors and the most refined flavors, berries belong to a very restricted class of foods whose place in the diet has much more to do with the passion we feel for their fragrance and delicacy than for their nutritional value. If you love berries, you will perhaps be surprised to learn that these delicious fruits are a veritable treasure chest of phytochemical compounds with anticancer potential. It just shows that what tastes good can also be good for health!

## Raspberries

It seems that the raspberry (from the earlier *raspis berry*, possibly from *raspis*, "a sweet rose-colored wine," or the Old French *raspe*, also meaning raspberry) has long been a much sought-after fruit, the gods of Olympus themselves having enjoyed this extraordinary tasting berry. So much so that to calm down the young Zeus, who suffered from dreadful fits punctuated by furious cries, Ida, the nymph who was his nursemaid, tried to pick a raspberry for him from the bramble bushes covering the Cretan mountainside where Zeus had been hidden from the murderous instincts of his terrible father Cronus. In so doing, she scratched her breast and her blood flowed onto the raspberries, which were white at the time, forever tinting them a brilliant scarlet. This extraordinary legend has been passed down through the centuries and, at the beginning of the first century, Pliny the

Elder still believed Mount Ida to be the only place where raspberries grew. Although it is likely that raspberry bushes originated in the mountainous regions of East Asia rather than in Greece, scientists nonetheless gave it the name of *Rubus idaeus*, or Ida's bramble, in homage to this charming story.

In addition to possessing undeniable taste qualities, raspberries have long played a role in the traditional medicine of many cultures, whether as an antidote used by the Russians, or to postpone aging, as used by the Chinese. Just like strawberries, raspberries contain large amounts of a very powerful anticancer molecule, ellagic acid, and are a fascinating food.

## Strawberries

The strawberry plant is a very resistant plant that grows wild in most regions of the world, both in the Americas and in Europe and Asia. Because of this, it is likely that the origin of eating wild strawberries is inseparable from the origin of human beings themselves, a fact attested to by the discovery of a great many strawberry seeds in prehistoric dwellings. Called *fraga* by the Romans because of its exquisite fragrance, the ancient strawberry (*Fragaria vesca*) grew exclusively in the underbrush. Oddly, the Romans did not really value its taste qualities

and, since Virgil wrote in *The Bucolics*, "Young people who gather budding flowers and fruits, flee this place; a cold snake lies in the grass," it is a safe bet that the pleasant meetings that took place during the gathering of these strawberries by young Roman men and women were more attractive than the strawberries!

It appears that strawberry cultivation began in France around the middle of the 14th century, following the efforts of gardeners to transplant wild strawberry plants into the royal gardens. Considerable efforts were made, definitely indicating a royal infatuation with these fruits since, in 1368, Jean Dudoy, then gardener to King Charles V, transplanted no fewer than 1,200 strawberry plants into the royal gardens at the Louvre in Paris. This close relationship between royalty and strawberries occurred several times in France's history — when Louis XIII went to Aquitaine in 1622 to quell the region's protestant rebellion, his meal consisted of strawberries in wine and sugar, as well as a strawberry cream pie.

The strawberry we know today is very different from the one consumed at that time and results from selections made from two varieties of strawberry plants different from those in Europe. At the beginning of the 17th century, French explorers brought back from their North American travels an interesting variety, the Scarlet Strawberry (*Fragaria virginiana*), which would be grown on a larger scale in the greenhouses at Versailles under Louis XIII and Louis XIV; the Sun King was so fond of strawberries that he could eat them to the point of indigestion. We owe the variety of strawberry eaten today all over the world to Amédée-François Frézier, whose name — similar to the French word for strawberry plant, *fraisier* — may have foreordained him to play a major role in the history of strawberries. An officer and cartographer in the French military, assigned in 1712 to observe the Spanish ports and plans for the fortification of the Western coast of South America, Frézier noticed on the Chilean coast a variety of strawberry plant with large white fruits, the Chilean white strawberry (*Fragaria chiloensis*). He successfully took five plants of this variety back to France, and while these plants did not bear fruit, their blooms

## Strawberry symbols and myths

While the origin of the strawberry is less poetic than that of the raspberry, several symbols, myths and legends are nonetheless associated with this berry. For some North American indigenous peoples, the souls of the dead can only forget the world of the living after having found and eaten a giant strawberry that sates their appetite and allows them to rest in peace for all eternity. For Westerners, the strawberry's red color, its tender flesh, its sweet juice and its resemblance to the heart have made it instead a synonym for temptation, as well as for love and sensuality.

Strawberries were also used long ago for beauty treatments, including fighting wrinkles and toning the skin. The seductive Madame Tallien, the ambassador of Paris fashion after the Revolution, regularly crushed 20 pounds (9 kg) of strawberries in her warm bath water to preserve the freshness and firmness of her skin, a shameless waste that led her to display herself at the Opera in a sleeveless white silk tunic, without undergarments!

The only dark side of the strawberry is that this fruit, like a number of foods (chocolate, bananas, tomatoes), often causes false food allergies due to its property of stimulating the release of histamine by the immune system, which results in a number of unpleasant symptoms like asthma or hives. These pseudo-allergies do not involve the formation of specific antibodies, however, and are not as serious as a real strawberry allergy, which remains rare in adults (less than 1 percent of all food allergies).

nonetheless made it possible to pollinate other species, especially *F. virginiana*. This cross-breeding gave birth to the ancestor of the strawberry now grown on every continent, *Fragaria ananassa*.

The use of strawberries, and of the strawberry plant in general, for therapeutic purposes appears to be very ancient. The Ojibwa, indigenous North Americans from southeastern Ontario, prepared strawberry leaf infusions to treat stomach upsets, as well as gastrointestinal disorders like diarrhea. But strawberries were not only well-known for their purgative properties; the famous Swedish botanist Linnaeus was convinced that an intensive course of treatment with strawberries was responsible for his miraculous recovery from a gout attack, and the French philosopher Fontanelle, who lived to be a hundred (1657–1757), attributed the secret of his longevity to his annual treatments, also based on strawberries. While we may find these anecdotes amusing, it is nonetheless true that recent scientific data indicate that strawberries might actually be an important food for cancer prevention.

## Blueberries and bilberries

A close relative of the European bilberry (*Vaccinium myrtillus*), the blueberry (*Vaccinium angustifolium*) is a species native to northeastern North America, where it has long been a part of the diet. Indigenous North Americans actually worshipped this fruit, which they believed sent by the gods to save their families from famine. Europeans newly arrived in North America quickly adopted the blueberry into their diet.

Indigenous North Americans prized the blueberry not only for food, but also for its medicinal properties. Among other things, they made an infusion from the plant's roots to relieve stress during pregnancy, as well as an infusion of the leaves to tone the body and reduce colic in children. The Algonquin really believed in blueberry's properties as a relaxant — they even served the plant's flowers to treat madness!

In the ancient world as well, bilberry cured several different common ailments like diarrhea, dysentery and scurvy. It has long been thought that this fruit has the ability to treat blood circulation disorders, as well as some eye diseases like diabetic retinopathies, glaucoma and cataracts, with these properties still being used by some doctors. This use is all the more interesting because we now know that diabetic retinopathies, for example, are diseases caused by the uncontrolled angiogenesis of retinal vessels, a process similar to that which supports tumor growth by means of the formation of a new blood vessel network (see Chapter 3). As we will see later, recent scientific data suggest that a class of molecules especially plentiful in blueberries and bilberries, the anthocyanidins, could be responsible for the antiangiogenic effects of these fruits and, as a result, help limit tumor growth.

## Cranberries

Despite their red color and their very tangy taste, cranberries are full members of the *Vaccinium* family and are as a result closely related to blueberries and bilberries. Just like the blueberry, the cranberry has a European cousin (*Vaccinium vitis idaea*), but the best-known varieties are those in North America, *Vaccinium oxycoccus* (little fruits) and *Vaccinium acrocarpon* (large fruits), with the latter being the variety now cultivated for commercial purposes.

As a general rule, cranberries play a relatively limited role in modern dietary habits, aside from being an accompaniment for turkey at Thanksgiving, a holiday celebrated in the United States that goes back to 1621. Indigenous North Americans, on the other hand, loved this fruit that they called "atoca"; they literally ate in it

every form imaginable, mainly dried as well as in a dish made of dried meat and fat prepared for the long winter months, called pemmican. Without a scientific understanding, indigenous peoples benefited from cranberries' high benzoic acid content, a natural agent that allowed food to be preserved longer. Nowadays, cranberries are often consumed as juice, which is a shame, since commercial juice contains large quantities of sugar and far fewer of the phytochemical molecules that give cranberries beneficial properties.

One of the best-known reasons to consume cranberries, in popular tradition, is to combat urinary infections. By watching indigenous North Americans use it to treat bladder and kidney disorders, settlers discovered this little fruit's

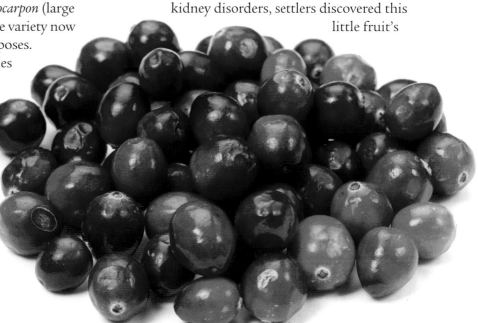

therapeutic effects. It is remarkable that this medicinal tradition again has a scientific basis, as it was later observed that some compounds in cranberries prevent bacteria from adhering to the cells of the urinary canal, thus reducing the risk of developing an infection in the tissue. As we will see later on, these molecules in cranberries, also found in blueberries, might also play a role in cancer prevention.

## The anticancer potential of berries: Ellagic acid, anthocyanidins and proanthocyanidins

Given that berries occupy a relatively limited space in the diet, since they are a seasonal fruit, only recently has their impact on cancer prevention been able to be examined. And the results obtained to date are very interesting, with the regular consumption of blueberries and strawberries being associated with a decline of about 30 percent in the risk of hormone-dependent breast cancer (ER-) (Figure 38, Chapter 5). This protection is not surprising, as researchers who are interested in the anticancer activity of various foods constantly mention berries as being important foods for cancer prevention. Let's look at why this is so.

### Ellagic acid

Of all the phytochemical compounds associated with berries, ellagic acid is without doubt the one most likely to interfere in cancer development. This molecule is an unusual-looking polyphenol (Figure 67) found mainly in raspberries and strawberries, as well as in some nuts like hazelnuts and pecans (Figure 68). However, even though raspberries appear at first glance to have a higher amount of ellagic acid than strawberries, we must bear in mind that 90 percent of the molecule in raspberries is in the seeds, whereas in strawberries 95 percent of it is in the flesh. It is therefore possible and even probable that the molecule in strawberries is more easily assimilated than that in raspberries. In this vein, it is interesting to note that the "Orleans," a variety of strawberry containing very high levels of ellagic acid (as well as other phytochemical compounds) was recently developed in Canada, which makes it likely the first "nutrapreventive" strawberry known to date.

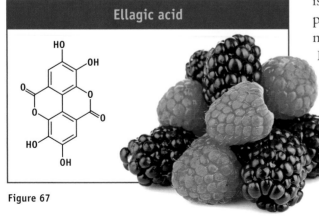

**Ellagic acid**

Figure 67

The anticancer potential of the main food sources of ellagic acid, that is, strawberries and raspberries, has been studied by means of cancer cells, as well as in laboratory animals subjected to a treatment causing cancer formation.

Strawberry extracts as well as raspberry extracts are able to thwart the growth of tumor cells, with these effects being directly connected to the quantity of polyphenols associated with fruits, but not to their antioxidant potential. In animals, studies have shown that a diet containing a relatively high proportion of strawberries or raspberries (5 percent of the diet) causes a significant reduction in the

number of tumors of the esophagus caused by NMBA, a powerful carcinogen. Similar results have been observed in humans after the administration of strawberry polyphenol extracts, suggesting that berries are a weapon of choice in the prevention of esophageal cancer.

The mechanisms by which ellagic acid interferes with cancer development at first glance resemble those we have described for a number of other foods. Currently available data indicate that ellagic acid prevents the activation of carcinogenic substances into cellular toxins; the latter thus lose their ability to react with DNA and to cause mutations that may trigger cancer. Ellagic acid also appears to increase cells' ability to defend themselves against toxic attack by stimulating their mechanisms for eliminating carcinogenic substances. That said, our own research results indicate that ellagic acid might be a more versatile anticancer molecule than was thought. We have discovered that this molecule is a powerful inhibitor of two proteins essential for tumor vascularization (VEGF and PDGF), the angiogenesis process described earlier (see Chapter 3). In fact, just as we observed for some of the components of green tea, ellagic acid is almost as powerful as some of the molecules developed by the pharmaceutical industry to interfere with cell activities leading to the formation of blood vessel networks in tumors. Given the importance of angiogenesis in the

### Ellagic acid content of various fruits and nuts

| Food | Ellagic acid (mg/portion)* |
| --- | --- |
| Raspberries (and blackberries) | 22 |
| Nuts | 20 |
| Pecans | 11 |
| Strawberries | 9 |
| Cranberries | 1.8 |
| Various fruits (blueberries, citrus fruits, peaches, kiwis, apples, pears, cherries) | Less than 1 |

* Serving of 5 ounces/150 g of fruit and 1 ounce/30 g of nuts

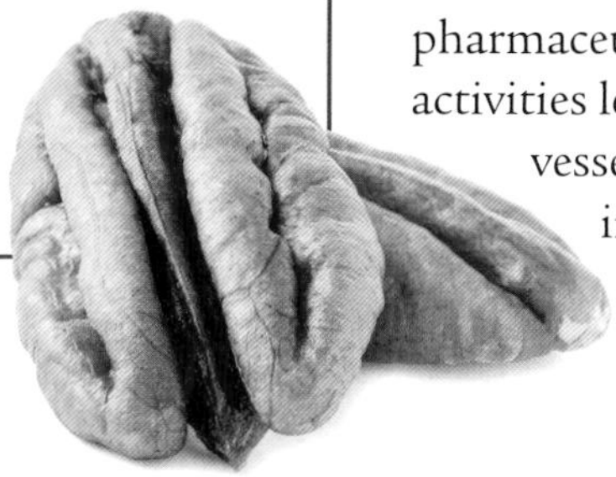

**Figure 68**

occurrence and progression of these tumors, it goes without saying that ellagic acid's antiangiogenic activity most certainly adds to its anticancer potential and, therefore, that strawberries and raspberries deserve special attention in any strategy for preventing cancer through diet.

*Anthocyanidins*

Anthocyanidins are a class of polyphenols responsible for the vast majority of the red, pink, purple, orange and blue colors of many fruits and vegetables. For example, an anthocyanidin called delphinidin (Figure 69) is responsible for the dark blue color of blueberries, while the cyanidin in cherries gives these fruits their characteristic red color. These pigments are especially plentiful in berries, which can contain up to 500 mg/100 g. In those who eat large amounts of these fruits, daily anthocyanidin intake may reach 200 mg, making them one of the most consumed groups of polyphenols.

According to some data, in addition to having high antioxidant activity, anthocyanidins may have a major impact on cancer development. For example, adding various anthocyanidins to cells isolated from tumors triggers an array of processes, such as the cessation of DNA synthesis and thus cell growth, leading to cell death by apoptosis. One of the anticancer effects of anthocyanidins also seems to be linked to angiogenesis inhibition. We have actually discovered that an anthocyanidin in blueberries, delphinidin, can inhibit the activity of the VEGF receptor associated with the development of angiogenesis, in concentrations close to those that can be attained though food. It is interesting to note that this activity is without doubt linked to delphinidin's antioxidant nature, as a very similar molecule found in large quantity in bilberries, malvidin, has an antioxidant activity identical to that of delphinidin, but shows no ability whatsoever to interfere with the receptor.

The anticancer potential of the anthocyanidins in blueberries and the ellagic acid in strawberries and raspberries suggests that including these fruits in the diet might have extraordinary repercussions for cancer prevention. While all berries contain large amounts of ellagic acid or anthocyanidins, we should note that black raspberries and blackberries are the only ones that contain both of these molecules. It is

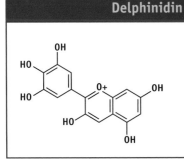

**Delphinidin**

**Figure 69**

therefore likely that these fruits may also prove to be valuable allies. In this vein, recent studies show that black raspberry extracts hinder the progression of esophageal cancer in animals and cause adenomatous polyps to regress in individuals at high risk for colon cancer (familial rectocolic polyposis).

*Proanthocyanidins*

Proanthocyanidins are complex polyphenols consisting of several units of the same molecule, catechins, forming a chain of variable length (Figure 70). These polymers can form complexes with proteins, especially the proteins in saliva, a property responsible for the astringency of foods containing these molecules. Although proanthocyanidins are plentiful in the seeds, flowers and bark of many plants, their presence in edible foods is quite limited (Figure 71). If we exclude cinnamon and cocoa, very significant sources but which cannot be consumed daily in large amounts (a debatable assertion in the eyes of some where cocoa is concerned), cranberries and blueberries are the best food sources of these molecules. The other berries discussed in this chapter contain much less of them, although strawberries' proanthocyanidin content makes

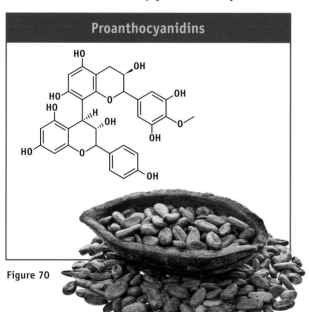

Figure 70

### Proanthocyanidins

| Proanthocyanidin content of various foods | |
| --- | --- |
| Foods | Proanthocyanidin content (mg/100 g) |
| Cinnamon | 8,108 |
| Cocoa powder | 1,373 |
| Red beans | 563 |
| Hazelnuts | 501 |
| Cranberries | 418 |
| Wild blueberries | 329 |
| Strawberries | 145 |
| Apples (Red Delicious) with peel | 128 |
| Grapes | 81 |
| Red wine | 62 |
| Raspberries | 30 |
| Cranberry juice | 13 |
| Grapeseed oil | 0 |

Figure 71

Source: USDA Database for the Proanthocyanidin Content of Selected Foods, 2004.

them stand out favorably in comparison with several other foods. On the other hand, it is important to note that cranberry juice contains far fewer proanthocyanidins that the fruit in its natural state and cannot therefore be considered a significant source of these molecules.

Proanthocyanidins are especially known as molecules with exceptional antioxidant power. An illustration of this occurred on Jacques Cartier's second voyage to North America, during which his crew, compelled to spend the winter in Canada, was especially hard hit by scurvy. As Cartier wrote in 1535 in his logbook, "The mouth became so disgusting and rotten because of the gums that almost all of the flesh fell off, right to the roots of the teeth, most of which fell out." Domagaya, an Iroquois who had accompanied Cartier to France on his first voyage, then showed him the secret of a herbal tea made from the bark and needles of a Canadian conifer believed to be the *Thuya occidentalis*, the Canadian white cedar. All of the sailors were quickly cured, and we now know that this miraculous recovery was related to the herbal tea's exceptional proanthocyanidin content, which successfully counteracted the effects of the lack of vitamin C.

In terms of cancer prevention, studies on the anticancer potential of proanthocyanidins are just beginning, but results obtained to date are encouraging. In the laboratory, adding these molecules inhibits the growth of some kinds of cancer cells, notably those derived from the colon, suggesting that proanthocyanidins might play a role in preventing the development of cancer. This agrees with some population studies showing that people who consume the highest amounts of proanthocyanidins have a lower risk of getting colon, stomach and prostate cancer. At the same time, it has been more and more clearly established that proanthocyanidins have the property of disrupting the development of new blood vessels through angiogenesis and might therefore help maintain microtumors in a latent state by preventing them from forming the blood vessels necessary for them to progress. Lastly, we should mention that studies indicate that some proanthocyanidins reduce estrogen synthesis and might therefore counteract the harmful effects of too high a level of these hormones. Even though the mechanisms responsible for these biological effects are still not understood, there is no doubt that proanthocyanidins have very intriguing characteristics from the perspective of cancer prevention and that introducing foods high in these molecules, like cranberries and chocolate (see Chapter 16), can only be beneficial.

Whether for their powerful antiangiogenic activity or their antioxidant properties, berries are an important source of anticancer phytochemical compounds and deserve a special place in a diet aiming to prevent cancer. And all the more so since introducing these delicious fruits into the daily diet should be popular with everyone!

## In summary:

- Berries are an excellent source of polyphenols with anticancer potential: ellagic acid, anthocyanidins and proanthocyanidins.

- It is preferable to consume dried cranberries rather than juice, by adding them to breakfast cereals or to dried fruit mixtures, for example.

- Blueberries and other berries can be frozen and eaten year-round, added to yogurt, ice cream or desserts.

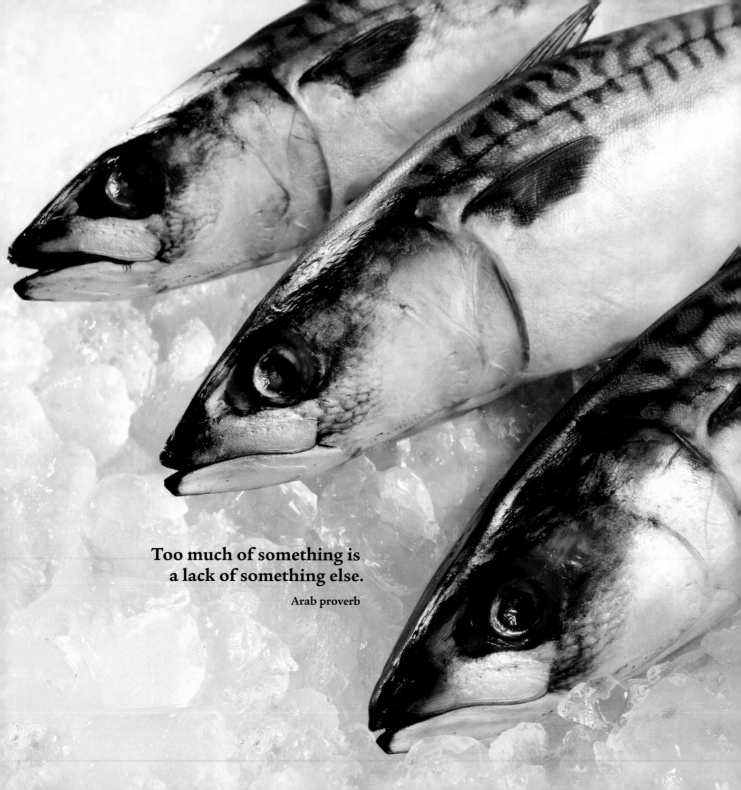

**Too much of something is
a lack of something else.**

Arab proverb

# Chapter 12

# Omega-3s: Finally, Fats that are Good for You!

In recent years, fats have gained a very bad reputation. While some fats, like "trans" fats, definitely deserve this negative opinion, there are some very good fats that actually have essential roles to play in the body's proper functioning (Figure 72). In other words, we must not only focus on the quantity of fats in the diet, but also on the quality of these fats. This is an important concept, for despite the great importance attached to fats in the Western diet, the largest nutritional deficiency among Westerners is paradoxically that of essential fatty acids, known as omega-3s.

## Essential fatty acids

Polyunsaturated fatty acids (omega-3 and omega-6) are said to be essential because the human body cannot produce them on its own, and they must therefore be supplied by food. For omega-6 fatty acids this requirement is not a problem, as these fats occur in large amounts in the modern diet's main components (meat, eggs, vegetables and various vegetable oils) and provide a sufficient supply of linoleic acid (LA), the most important fat in this category.

The situation with regard to omega-3 fatty acids is more complex, since these fats are much less widely distributed in nature. There

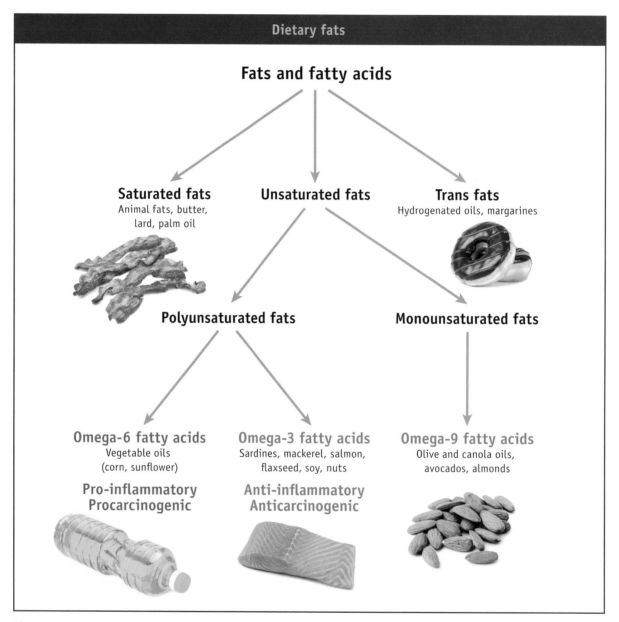

## Dietary fats

**Fats and fatty acids**

**Saturated fats**
Animal fats, butter,
lard, palm oil

**Unsaturated fats**

**Trans fats**
Hydrogenated oils, margarines

**Polyunsaturated fats**

**Monounsaturated fats**

**Omega-6 fatty acids**
Vegetable oils
(corn, sunflower)

**Pro-inflammatory
Procarcinogenic**

**Omega-3 fatty acids**
Sardines, mackerel, salmon,
flaxseed, soy, nuts

**Anti-inflammatory
Anticarcinogenic**

**Omega-9 fatty acids**
Olive and canola oils,
avocados, almonds

**Figure 72**

are two major types of omega-3s: linolenic acid (LNA), a short-chain omega-3 fatty acid found in plants, mainly in flaxseeds and some nuts (especially walnuts); and docosahexaenoic (DHA) and eicosapentaenoic (EPA) acids, long-chain omega-3s found almost exclusively in fatty fish (Figure 73). Plant LNA can be partially transformed into DHA and EPA inside our cells,

| Main dietary sources of omega-3 fatty acids | |
|---|---|
| **Plant sources** | **Linolenic acid content (LNA)** (g/serving)* |
| Fresh walnuts | 2.6 |
| Flaxseed | 2.2 |
| Walnut oil | 1.4 |
| Canola oil | 1.3 |
| Soybeans | 0.44 |
| Tofu | 0.26 |
| **Animal sources** | **EPA and DHA content** (g/serving)* |
| Sardines | 2.0 |
| Herring | 2.0 |
| Mackerel | 1.8 |
| Salmon (Atlantic) | 1.6 |
| Rainbow trout | 1.0 |

*1 tablespoon/15 ml serving of oils, 1 ounce/30 g of nuts and 3.5 ounces/100 g of tofu, beans and fish. Taken from the USDA Nutrient Data Laboratory (www.nal.usda.gov/fnic/foodcomp) and from tufts.edu/med/nutrition.

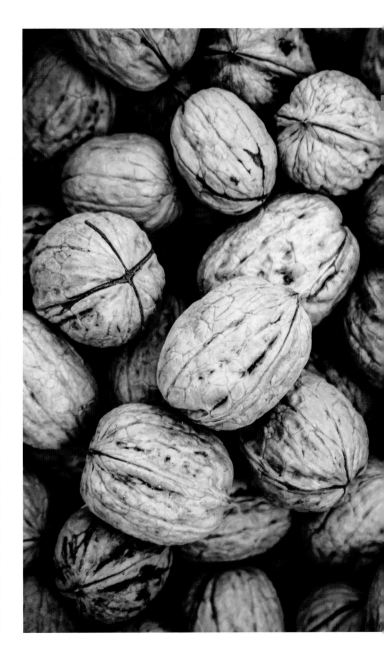

**Figure 73**

# What are we to make of all these fats?

The terminology of fats is admittedly not easy to grasp. Here are a few definitions that should help you better understand what terms like *saturated fats, polyunsaturated fats, "trans" fats* and *omega-3 fatty acids* actually mean.

Fatty acids can be compared to chains of varying lengths whose rigidity fluctuates depending on various parameters (Figure 74). *Saturated* fats have straight chains in which molecules are pressed tightly together and are therefore more stable. This is why butter and animal fats, sources high in saturated fats, are solid at room temperature and in the refrigerator.

*Polyunsaturated* fatty acids have a different structure. Their chains have bends that are rigid in places, which means the molecules cannot be bound together as tightly and are thus more flexible, a property that makes vegetable oils liquid, for example.

*Monounsaturated* fatty acids fall somewhere between the two, as their chains have only a single rigid point. This is why olive oil, a source high in these fats, is liquid at room temperature but solidifies in the refrigerator.

The properties of fatty acids can be modified, however. If polyunsaturated fatty acids are *hydrogenated* using industrial methods, their rigid points are destroyed and their chains lose their structure. They then become solid at room temperature, as in the case of margarine. Unfortunately, this reaction causes modifications in the fatty acid structure, changing the layout of the chain; this is what we mean by *"trans" fat*, fats that very rarely occur naturally and can damage cells.

The term "omega," more and more fashionable in recent years, comes from the way scientists identify the location of the first rigid point on the fatty acid chain. These locations are numbered beginning at the end of the chain. Thus, a polyunsaturated omega-3 or omega-6 fatty acid is a fat whose first rigid point is at position 3 or 6. For the same reason, monounsaturated fatty acids are sometimes called omega-9, because the only rigid point in their chain occurs at position 9.

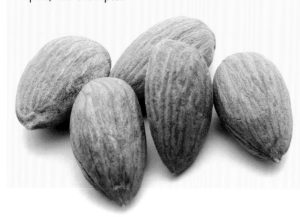

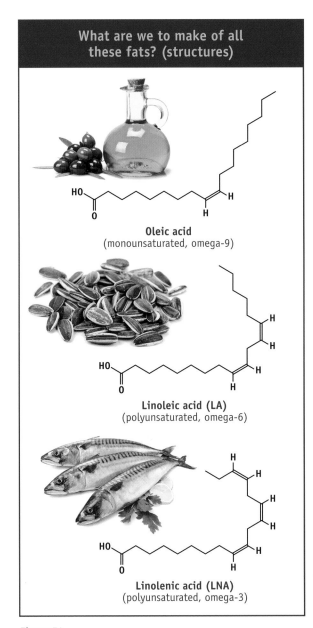

## What are we to make of all these fats? (structures)

**Oleic acid**
(monounsaturated, omega-9)

**Linoleic acid (LA)**
(polyunsaturated, omega-6)

**Linolenic acid (LNA)**
(polyunsaturated, omega-3)

**Figure 74**

but it seems that this conversion is not very effective in humans, especially when omega-6 fatty acids are overrepresented in the diet, as is the case today. In fact, when we consider that the proportion of omega-6/omega-3 fatty acids provided by the diet of the first human beings was roughly equal, likely in the neighborhood of 1:1, this ratio is now estimated to be 20:1, and even higher in people who regularly consume industrially processed food products.

The difficulty in producing EPA and DHA is due to the fact that the enzyme machinery that makes these acids from LNA also transforms LA, or omega-6, into inflammatory molecules like prostaglandins. Thus, when the diet provides too much LA, these enzymes become submerged in the excess fat and simply cannot effectively recognize the LNA present in lower amounts. This imbalance in favor of omega-6s may have negative repercussions and encourage the development of chronic diseases like heart disease and cancer, since the omega-6s are used by the body to produce molecules that promote inflammation, whereas omega-3s are essential for the production of anti-inflammatory molecules (Figure 75). Increasing omega-3 intake and decreasing the amount of omega-6 could thus significantly reduce risk for all inflammatory diseases, heart disease as well as cancer.

One good way to lower omega-6 fatty acid intake is to use olive oil as your main fat source (canola oil is also an option owing to

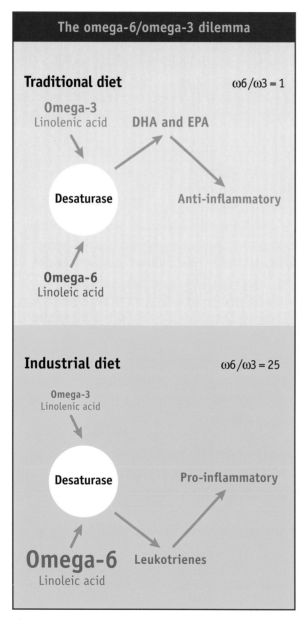

**The omega-6/omega-3 dilemma**

**Traditional diet**  ω6/ω3 = 1

**Omega-3**
Linolenic acid

**DHA and EPA**

Desaturase

**Anti-inflammatory**

**Omega-6**
Linoleic acid

**Industrial diet**  ω6/ω3 = 25

**Omega-3**
Linolenic acid

Desaturase

**Pro-inflammatory**

**Omega-6**
Linoleic acid

**Leukotrienes**

**Figure 75**

its better omega-6/omega-3 ratio); this change has even more health benefits, as several recent observations indicate that olive oil has an anticancer action owing to its content of a number of polyphenols that reduce inflammation, kill cancer cells and hinder the formation of a blood vessel network through the process of angiogenesis (see box).

Increasing omega-3 intake is really just a matter of incorporating as many vegetable sources as possible – like flaxseeds or nuts – into the diet and regularly eating fatty fish (sardines, mackerel, salmon) containing high levels of DHA and EPA already present and ready for cells to use.

## The beneficial effects of omega-3 fatty acids

The importance of increasing our intake of omega-3 fats stems from their many positive roles in ensuring our body functions properly. DHA and EPA are absolutely essential for the development of the brain and retinal cells during pregnancy, they play a crucial role in the transmission of nerve impulses by promoting better communication among brain cells, and their presence in the membrane of heart cells maintains a regular heartbeat and thus prevents the episodes of arrhythmia that are often precursors of embolisms or sudden death.

# Cancer cells hate olive oil!

People who follow a Mediterranean-style diet have roughly 15 percent less risk of getting cancer, a protection that might even be as high as 60 percent for some cancers, like uterine or breast cancer. Several recent studies have emphasized, among the factors that contribute to this protective effect, the leading role played by the antioxidant and anti-inflammatory phenolic compounds in olive oil. For example, this oil contains significant quantities (0.2 mg/ml) of a molecule called oleocanthal, which has an anti-inflammatory activity similar to ibuprofen and might thus have effects similar to this molecule in preventing colon cancer. Oleocanthal can also kill a wide range of cancer cells very rapidly (in less than 30 minutes), a property that derives from its ability to force cells to "digest themselves." Work in our laboratory has also shown that other phenolic compounds in olive oil (hydroxytyrosol, taxifolin) block the activity of a receptor (VEGFR2) essential to the formation of new blood vessels in tumors and could therefore hinder the occurrence and growth of a large number of cancers. The presence of all of these molecules means that olive oil can be considered the only fat with anticancer activity.

It is important to choose virgin or extra-virgin olive oil, since these oils are cold-pressed (below 81°F/27°C) and contain the polyphenols from the olives.

It is actually quite easy to check for these phenolic compounds: oleocanthal, for example, has the odd property of interacting with a receptor located almost exclusively in the throat, which causes a tingling sensation typical of high-quality olive oils. The more it tingles, the higher the oleocanthal content and the better the olive oil's anticancer action!

One of the most important roles of omega-3s, however, remains their powerful anti-inflammatory action. Several mechanisms are at play. For example, omega-3s from plants (linolenic acid) prevent the synthesis of enzymes responsible for producing inflammatory molecules (COX-2), as well as certain molecules that initiate inflammation (IL-6, TNF); omega-3s from animal sources (DHA and EPA) are natural anti-inflammatory molecules that prevent the immune system from overreacting and damaging tissues. These properties mean that a diet containing large quantities of these molecules prevents the creation of a state of chronic inflammation in the body and thus reduces the development of diseases that depend on this inflammation to progress.

The first evidence of the benefits of a diet high in omega-3 fatty acids comes from studies that have shown that, despite a diet exclusively based on an intake of very fatty meats (seal, whale, etc.) and lacking in fruits and vegetables, the Inuit of Greenland are largely free of cardiovascular diseases. This protection is not genetic, for when they emigrate the Inuit become subject to these diseases; it is apparently related to the exceptional omega-3 fatty acid content of the seafood they consume. Several subsequent studies have confirmed that eating fish high in omega-3 does in fact help prevent heart disease by lowering the risk of cardiac arrhythmia, the main cause of sudden death. As a result, organizations fighting heart disease, like the American Heart Association, recommend eating at least two meals a week of fatty fish to lower the risk of these diseases.

Nor should the importance of plant-sourced omega-3s be ignored: in recent years, several studies have clearly shown that simply eating three servings of nuts a week is enough to reduce by 40 to 60 percent the mortality risk associated with heart

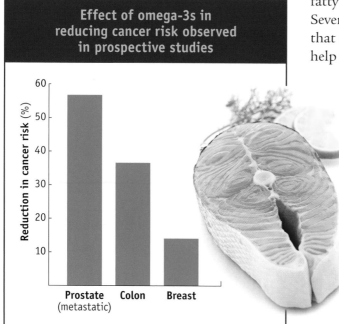

**Effect of omega-3s in reducing cancer risk observed in prospective studies**

Reduction in cancer risk (%)

Prostate (metastatic)  Colon  Breast

Figure 76

disease and by 20 percent to 40 percent the mortality from cancer. Flaxseeds are another outstanding source of omega-3 that can have positive effects on cancer risk, both for its LNA and its phytoestrogen content. Just two tablespoons of flaxseeds provide more than 140 percent of the daily recommended intake of omega-3!

*Omega-3 and cancer*

The health benefits of omega-3s are not limited to heart disease, however; more and more experimental results suggest that fatty acids may also play a role in cancer prevention. For example, a number of studies designed to examine the relationship between the consumption of fish high in omega-3 and cancer have shown a reduction in the risk of developing breast, colon and prostate cancer (the metastatic form of the disease) (Figure 76), as well as a high survival rate for these cancers. A reduction in uterine cancer risk and liver cancer risk has also been suggested, but this requires further study. The positive impact of omega-3s on prostate cancer seems to be especially linked to the inhibition of the progression of tumor microfoci in advanced cancer, with a 63 percent reduction in mortality associated with this disease in some studies.

It is interesting to note that plant sources of omega-3 like nuts also seem to have anticancer effects: for example, one study done on 75,680 women showed that those who ate a serving of nuts (1 ounce/28 g) twice a week had a 35 percent lower risk of getting pancreatic cancer than those who never ate nuts.

The role of omega-3 fatty acids in the prevention of some types of cancer is borne out by results obtained using animal models and isolated tumor cells. For example, while omega-6 fatty acids are known to be factors that trigger cancer, introducing omega-3s into the food of laboratory rats causes the opposite effect; they reduce the development of breast, colon, prostate and pancreatic cancers, and increase the effectiveness of chemotherapy drugs. The mechanism involved in these protective effects could be linked to a drop in the production of inflammatory molecules that damage the immune system and promote cancer development, as well as to a direct effect on cancer cells, by modifying their ability to avoid death by apoptosis and by preventing the development of new blood vessels required for their growth. Thus, increased consumption of foods high in omega-3s, like fatty fish, especially if they replace saturated animal fats like red meat, can only be good for health and help reduce significantly the risk of cancer.

In short, there is absolutely no doubt that changing our diet by consuming significantly more omega-3 fatty acids and fewer omega-6 fatty acids can have a preventive effect against cancer. A tablespoon of freshly ground flaxseeds added to cereals in the morning is a simple and effective way to increase omega-3 intake. However, do not use seeds already ground; instead buy whole seeds you can grind at home. This will retain all the goodness of their essential fats.

Since the best source of these fats is fish, everything points to incorporating two or three servings of fatty fish into your weekly diet, both for their omega-3 content and their exemplary protein, vitamin and mineral content. It is obviously a shame that some fish contain tiny amounts of various toxic substances, but remember that in such small quantities the benefits fish provides are far greater than the negative effects of these substances. If however this is a concern for you, avoid eating large predatory fish like shark, swordfish and tuna more than once a week. Those fish that are good sources of omega-3 (salmon, sardines, mackerel) only contain trace amounts of toxic substances.

**In summary:**

- Currently, the biggest nutritional deficiency in Western countries is the low intake of omega-3 polyunsaturated fatty acids.

- Since omega-3s are by nature extremely unstable, it is better to use whole foods as a source of these fats rather than omega-3 supplements.

- Eating fatty fish once or twice a week is a simple way to increase the amount of omega-3s in the diet. Similarly, freshly ground flaxseeds stored in a sealed container in the refrigerator can be added to breakfast cereals.

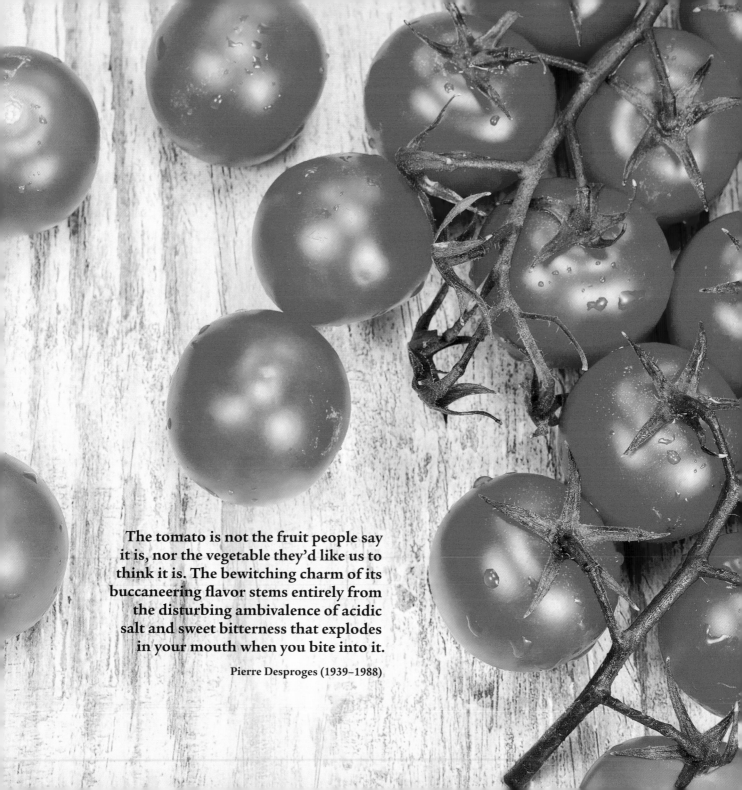

The tomato is not the fruit people say
it is, nor the vegetable they'd like us to
think it is. The bewitching charm of its
buccaneering flavor stems entirely from
the disturbing ambivalence of acidic
salt and sweet bitterness that explodes
in your mouth when you bite into it.

Pierre Desproges (1939–1988)

# Chapter 13

# Tomatoes: Turning Cancer Red with Shame

Tomatoes originated in South America, very likely Peru, where they are actually still found in the wild. Yellow in color and the size of today's cherry tomatoes, these Peruvian tomatoes were not eaten by the Incas, however. It was instead the Aztecs of Central America who began to cultivate what they called *tomalt*, the "plump fruit" that they were already combining with chili peppers to make what was doubtless the ancestor of what we now know as salsa.

Discovered by the Spanish during the conquest of Mexico at the beginning of the 16th century, the tomato first appeared in Spain, and then in Italy, where by 1544 the resemblance of this *pomo d'oro* to belladonna and the fearsome mandrake, two plants with very potent psychotropic effects, had already been noticed. That was enough to make people think tomatoes were a poisonous fruit, and for a long time they were only used as ornamental plants in northern Europe, to "cover cabinets and arbours, gaily climbing over them, attaching themselves firmly to supports [...]. Their fruit is not good to eat: they are only useful in medicine and pleasant to touch, to smell" (Olivier de Serres, *The Theatre of Agriculture*, 1600). It was not until

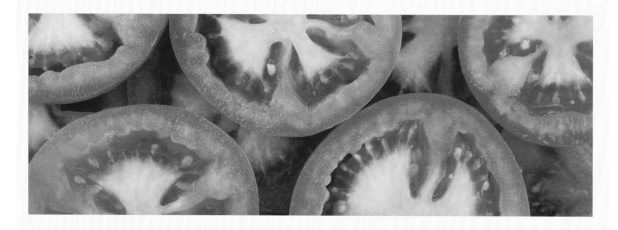

## Tomatoes: Fruit, vegetable or poison?

We may smile at ancient beliefs that tomatoes were dangerous to health, but we must nonetheless pay homage to their sense of observation: the tomato does indeed belong to a plant family — the Solanaceae — that includes several plants containing extremely powerful alkaloids that can even cause death, like tobacco, belladonna, mandrake and datura. Tomato plants actually contain one of these substances, tomatin, but it is found almost exclusively in the roots and leaves, with less in the fruit, and it disappears completely as the fruit ripens (this is also true of other edible Solanaceae like potatoes, eggplants and bell peppers). People's ambivalence toward tomatoes is well summed up by its botanical name, *Lycopersican esculentum*, which translates as "edible wolf peach," inspired by a German legend according to which witches used hallucinogenic plants like belladonna and mandrake to create werewolves.

Finally, note that the tomato can be considered both a fruit and a vegetable. From a botanical point of view, it is a fruit (actually a berry), since it results from the fertilization of a flower. But from a horticultural point of view, like squash, it is viewed as a vegetable, both because of its cultivation and its use. This classification is mainly economic: an American businessman wishing to be exempted from the taxes applied to vegetable imports tried to assert that the tomato was a fruit, a request rejected in 1893 by the American Supreme Court, which officially ruled the tomato a vegetable.

1692 that tomatoes first appeared in an Italian recipe book, and it would be another century before their culinary use would really begin to spread to the rest of Europe. The inhabitants of the New World were equally hesitant about including tomatoes in their daily diet, despite the example set by famous people, notably Thomas Jefferson, and they only came into common use around the middle of the 19th century. Today, tomatoes are one of the main sources of vitamins and minerals in the Western diet.

| Main dietary sources of lycopene | |
|---|---|
| **Food** | **Lycopene content** (mg/100 g) |
| Tomato paste | 29.3 |
| Tomato puree | 17.5 |
| Ketchup | 17 |
| Tomato sauce | 15.9 |
| Condensed tomato soup | 10.9 |
| Canned tomatoes | 9.7 |
| Tomato juice | 9.3 |
| Guava | 5.4 |
| Watermelon | 4.8 |
| Tomato (raw) | 3 |
| Papaya | 2 |
| Pink grapefruit | 1.5 |

**Figure 77**    Source: USDA Database for the Carotenoid Content of Selected Foods, 1998.

## Lycopene, the driving force behind tomatoes' anticancer properties

Lycopene belongs to the carotenoid family, a very varied class of phytochemical molecules that give many fruits and vegetables their yellow, orange and red color. Since the human body cannot produce carotenoids, these molecules must be obtained by including vegetables in the diet. Some carotenoids, like beta-carotene and beta-cryptoxanthin, are precursors of vitamin A, a vitamin essential for growth, while other members of this family, like lutein, zeaxanthin and lycopene, have no chemical effect related to vitamin A and therefore play different roles. For example, lutein and zeaxanthin absorb the blue in light very effectively and might therefore protect the eyes by reducing the risk of macular degeneration related to aging, as well as the formation of cataracts. The role of lycopene is still not well understood, but several recent observations suggest that, of all the carotenoids, it could be the one with the greatest impact on cancer prevention.

Lycopene is the pigment that gives tomatoes their red color, and this fruit-vegetable is by far its best dietary source. Generally speaking, tomato-based products provide about 85 percent of lycopene intake, with the other 15 percent coming from certain fruits (Figure 77). The lycopene content of our cultivated tomatoes is much lower than

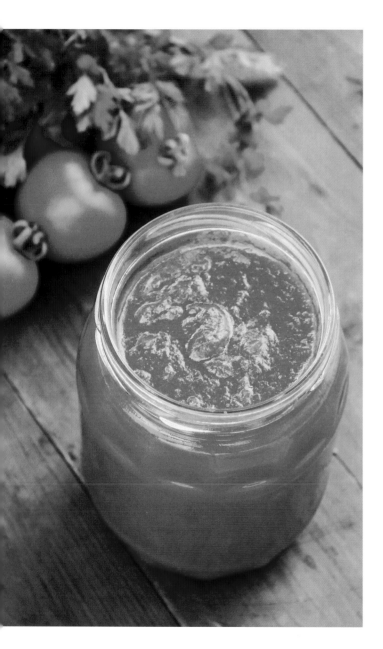

that of the original wild species, *Lycopersicon pimpinellifolium* (50 $\mu g$/g, compared with 200–250 $\mu g$ in some wild species). This difference can be explained by the limited number of species used for hybridization, which reduces the variability of the plant's genes. It is to be hoped that reintroducing genetic information from wild species will increase this level, so that lycopene levels even more likely to have an influence on cancer development can be reached.

Products made from cooked tomatoes are especially high in lycopene and, even more important, breaking down the cells with heat makes it easier to extract the molecule and causes changes to its structure (isomerization) that make it more easily absorbed by the body. Fats also increase lycopene's availability; when tomatoes are cooked in olive oil, the amount of lycopene that can be absorbed is maximized. Finally, in spite of what President Reagan's administration claimed in 1981 to justify its budget cutbacks in school cafeteria programs, ketchup is not a vegetable and its high lycopene content should not make us forget that almost two-thirds of its weight is sugar.

Countries where large amounts of tomatoes are consumed, like Italy, Spain and Mexico, have prostate cancer levels much lower than those in North America. Obviously, these statistics do not prove that the differences are connected to the role played by tomatoes in the diet (Asians do not eat tomatoes and are not especially affected by this disease), but they have nonetheless led researchers to try to establish a link between prostate cancer development and dietary intake of tomatoes. There are a number of studies suggesting that people who consume large quantities of tomatoes and tomato-based products have a lower risk of developing prostate cancer, especially the most invasive forms of this disease. For example, in studies on large population samples in which the risk of developing prostate cancer is correlated with

the consumption of foods high in lycopene, like tomato sauce, a decrease in risk of about 35 percent can be observed. This association appears to be stronger for men aged 65 and over, which indicates that lycopene is better at counteracting prostate cancer development associated with aging than that occurring earlier, around age 50, which seems to be genetic in origin.

The mechanisms by which lycopene reduces prostate cancer development are still unknown. Just like its close relative, beta-carotene, lycopene is an excellent antioxidant, but it is still not clear how this property contributes to its anticancer effect. In fact, according to results obtained to date, lycopene might impede prostate cancer development more by its direct action on some of the enzymes responsible for tissue growth, notably by interfering with signals from androgens, the hormones often involved in the excess growth of prostatic tissue, as well as by disturbing the growth of tissue cells. Since the lycopene absorbed tends to accumulate in the prostate, the molecule would thus be ideally located to prevent the possible excessive growth of cancer cells. However, although most research to date into the anticancer effect of tomatoes has mainly concentrated on the prevention of prostate cancer, several studies suggest that this fruit-vegetable could play a broader role in preventing other cancers, especially those

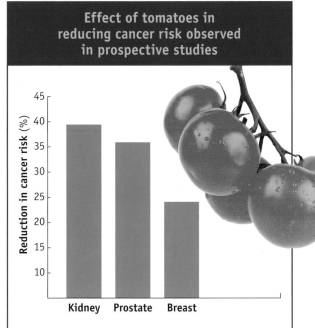

**Effect of tomatoes in reducing cancer risk observed in prospective studies**

Reduction in cancer risk (%)

Kidney  Prostate  Breast

Figure 78

of the kidney and breast (Figure 78). In the latter case, studies done on breast cancer cells in animal models show that lycopene blocks the proliferation of these cells, possibly by interfering with the action of sex hormones and certain growth factors.

It is also interesting to note that lycopene accumulates in the skin, where it can neutralize free radicals produced by the action of UV rays, thus helping to slow down skin aging and lower the risk of melanoma. The effect is long lasting, as biopsies taken from the lumbar region have shown that lycopene was still detectable four days after being ingested, remained in high concentrations in the skin for at least a week, and was still there 42 days later! These observations agree with some studies indicating that daily consumption of tomato paste is associated with a higher degree of skin protection against the sun, as well as a significant increase in collagen levels, two factors crucial for maintaining the skin's integrity. So it seems we can assume that lycopene is a multipurpose anticancer molecule able to interfere with the development of several different types of cancer. Tomatoes must therefore be considered a food that is part of a broader strategy for preventing cancer through diet.

Eating tomato-based products is a good way to lower the risk of getting prostate cancer. However, research results obtained to date indicate that the amount of lycopene required to see a significant decrease in risk is quite high. It is therefore important to choose products not only high in lycopene, but also in which the form of lycopene present is the one most easily absorbed by the body. Given this, tomato sauce is the ideal food, as it contains a high concentration of this molecule that is easily absorbed because the tomatoes are cooked for a long time in olive oil. Just eating two meals a week based on these sauces can reduce your risk of developing prostate cancer by 30 percent. And don't forget the garlic!

**In summary:**

- Lycopene, the pigment that gives tomatoes their red color, is the essential compound behind tomatoes' anticancer potential.

- Lycopene's anticancer action is however only maximized if the tomatoes are cooked in fat, like sauces made with tomato paste.

So, when you hold the hemisphere of a cut of lemon above your plate, you spill a universe of gold, a yellow goblet of miracles... the minute fire of a planet.

Pablo Neruda, "Ode to a Lemon," in *Elemental Odes* (1954)

# Chapter 14

# Citrus Fruit: Anticancer Molecules with Zest

Citrus fruits belong to the genus *Citrus*, comprising such sour-tasting and acidic fruits as lemons, oranges, grapefruit and mandarins (see box, pp. 192–193). They are also known botanically as *hesperidia*, referring to the 11th labor of Hercules, during which the demigod succeeded in picking golden apples from the garden guarded by the Hesperides nymphs. Nowadays, however, the name *hesperidia* is mainly used in perfumery to designate the essential oils obtained from plants in the genus *Citrus*.

All citrus fruits come originally from Asia, especially India and China, where they were cultivated at least 3,000 years ago. As a result, not until explorers made their way to and from the Asian continent did the first citrus fruits appear in the West: citron (*Citrus medica*), brought back by Alexander the Great in the fourth century BCE; bitter orange trees, introduced by the Arabs at the beginning of our era; and, much later, lemon trees, planted in Spain in the 12th century, orange trees in Portugal in the 15th century and, even more recently, mandarin trees in Provence and in North Africa in the 19th century. Long considered to be exotic fruits, citrus fruits are now part of the diet in the vast majority of countries, with a billion citrus trees cultivated worldwide, producing nearly 100 million tons of fruit each year.

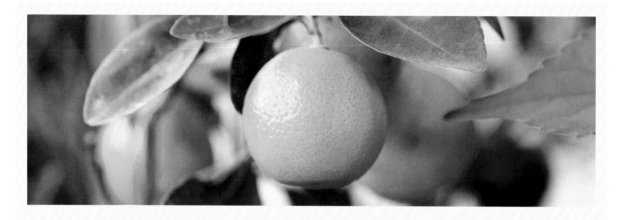

# The main citrus fruits

### Oranges (*Citrus sinensis*)

Although this fruit originated in China, the word "orange" appears to come from the Arabic *narandj*, in turn derived from the Sanskrit *nagarunga*, meaning "fruit loved by elephants." Sweet oranges were introduced in the West by the Portuguese, who began to cultivate them with considerable success and thus contributed greatly to making them popular. It was Christopher Columbus who, on his second voyage, took along the seeds that would give rise to the cultivation of orange trees in North America. Louis XIV, who loved oranges as much as strawberries, ordered that the famous orangeries be built at Versailles. Still deemed a luxury food at the beginning of the 20th century, the orange has become, since the Second World War, the most popular citrus fruit in the world and represents as much as 70 percent of worldwide citrus fruit production.

### Grapefruit (*Citrus paradisi Macfadyen*)

The grapefruit we know today is really a variety of pomelo created by crossing oranges and … grapefruit! In fact, the true grapefruit (*C. grandis*) gets its name from the Dutch *pompelmoes*, meaning "large lemon," a name given to a large pear-shaped fruit brought from Malaysia by the Dutch in the 17th century. What are sold as pomelos are actually grapefruits, whereas our grapefruits are really pomelos!

## Lemons (*Citrus limon*)

Likely originating in China or India, close to the Himalayas, the lemon was introduced in Europe in the 12th century by the Arabs. Lemons must not be confused with citrons, a fruit that had been brought to the Mediterranean by Alexander the Great and which, according to the writings of Theophrastus, Democrites and Virgil, was frequently used as an antidote. Lemons were soon used as a remedy to fight scurvy, but it was not until the 15th century that they really became an established part of European culinary habits. Despite their appearance and similar culinary use, limes (*Citrus aurantifolia*) are a different botanical species native to Malaysia and requiring a more tropical climate than lemons do to bear fruit.

## Mandarins (*Citrus reticula*)

Mandarins, whose name no doubt comes from the similarity of their color to the silk robes worn by Chinese mandarins, also originated in Southeast Asia and were likely domesticated 2,500 years ago in China. Grown on the shores of the Mediterranean since the 19th century, they have seen their popularity increase thanks to the development of their most famous hybrid, the clementine, in 1902. Today, mandarins, tangerines and clementines make up 10 percent of all of the citrus fruit produced worldwide.

## The phytochemical compounds in citrus fruit

Much more than a plentiful source of vitamin C, citrus fruits contain many phytochemical compounds responsible for their anticancer properties. For example, one orange contains almost 200 different compounds, including about 60 polyphenols, as well as several members of a class of very fragrant molecules called terpenes.

Citrus fruits are the only plants that contain large quantities of a group of polyphenols called flavanones, molecules that actively contribute to the antiscurvy effects long associated with these fruits. One of these molecules, hesperidin, was once even called "vitamin P," for its role in preserving blood vessel integrity by toning the vessels and making them less permeable. Since inflammatory processes are characterized by an

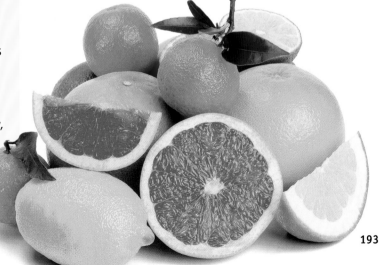

increase in blood vessel permeability, the effect of citrus fruit polyphenols really turns them into anti-inflammatory molecules that may help prevent cancer.

## The anticancer properties of citrus fruit

Studies done in different parts of the world have highlighted a link between consuming citrus fruit and a decrease in the risk of getting certain cancers; this relationship is especially convincing in the case of cancers of the digestive tract — the mouth, esophagus and stomach — where reductions of 40 percent to 50 percent have been observed (Figure 79). It is likely, however, that citrus fruit may also target other cancers, as an analysis of the food habits of 42,470 Japanese aged from 40 to 79 shows that people who consume citrus fruit daily have a 38 percent lower risk of getting cancers of the pancreas and prostate. Some studies also indicate that children who drink orange juice regularly in the first two years of their lives have a lower risk of getting leukemia later on. These encouraging results remain to be confirmed, but they bear witness once again to the impact that the composition of the diet can have on the development of some cancers, even in childhood.

In many respects, these observations are consistent with laboratory experiments, in which the main components of citrus fruits, polyphenols and terpenes, have often been identified as molecules able to interfere with processes responsible for cancer development. Although the mechanisms involved still remain largely unknown, some data suggest that the phytochemical compounds in citrus fruits block tumor growth by acting directly on cancer cells, reducing their ability to reproduce.

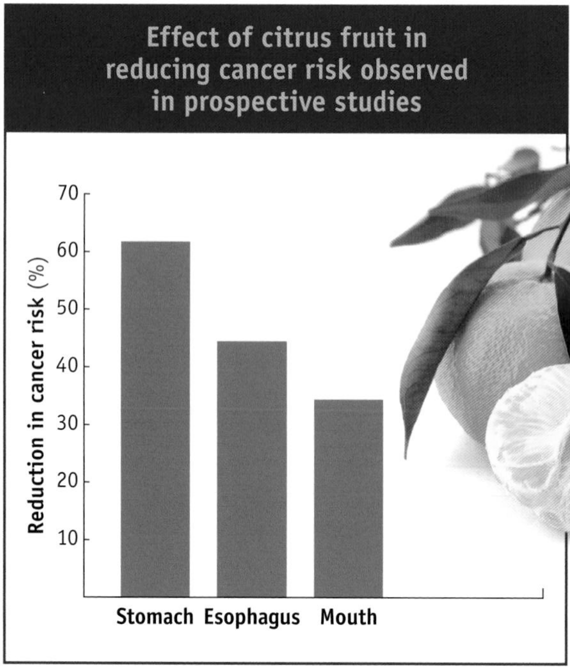

**Effect of citrus fruit in reducing cancer risk observed in prospective studies**

Figure 79

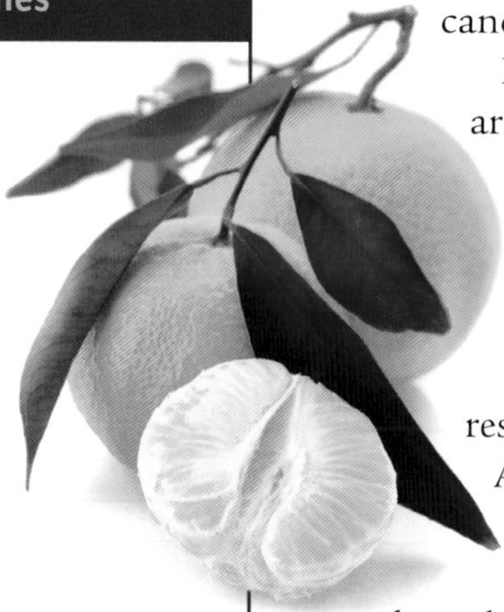

It is likely, however, that one of the main anticancer effects of citrus fruit is linked to their modulation of the detoxification systems of carcinogenic substances. The interaction of citrus fruit with these systems is clearly illustrated by the surprising effect that grapefruit juice can have on how some drugs are metabolized. In fact, in a study attempting to determine the impact of alcohol on the effectiveness of a drug commonly used to control cardiac arrhythmias, it was recognized quite by accident that the grapefruit juice used to mask the taste of alcohol caused the amount of the drug in the blood to double, in turn increasing the side effects. A similar effect has been observed in the case of statins, drugs used to reduce blood cholesterol. These observations show the degree to which citrus fruit can modulate the systems involved in the metabolism of foreign substances. We now know that these effects are due in large part to molecules belonging to the coumarin class (bergamottin and 6',7'-dihydroxybergamottin), which block an enzyme in the liver responsible for metabolizing drugs (cytochrome P4503A4). The fact that molecules associated with citrus fruit behave in this way is significant and may even prove crucial for maximizing the anticancer potential of other fruits and vegetables, since all the anticancer molecules in food that we have

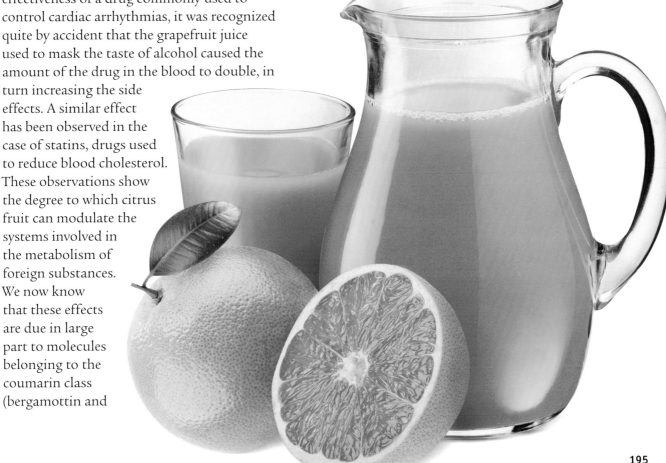

described in this book are transformed and eliminated from our body by the same enzyme systems as those involved in drug metabolism. In other words, inhibiting these systems by means of the phytochemical compounds in citrus fruit has the immediate consequence of slowing down this metabolism and considerably increasing the concentrations of anticancer compounds in the blood, thus making them more potent.

In conclusion, citrus fruits must not be thought of only as an excellent source of vitamin C, but also as foods able to supply the body with numerous anticancer phytochemical compounds. The many compounds in these fruits may not only act directly on cancer cells and thus prevent their progression, but also play a beneficial role by acting as anti-inflammatories and modifying the absorption and elimination of many substances. Consuming citrus fruit daily, preferably in the form of whole fruit, is therefore a simple and effective way to add "zesty freshness" to a cancer prevention diet.

**In summary:**

- Citrus fruits are foods essential for cancer prevention, because of both their direct action on cancer cells and their ability to enhance the anticancer potential of other phytochemical compounds in the diet.

- Consuming citrus fruit guarantees an incomparable source of these anticancer molecules, while at the same time providing the required daily amounts of several vitamins and minerals.

- It is preferable to consume these fruits in their whole form, as the high sugar content of some citrus fruits, along with a lack of fiber, can cause sudden fluctuations in blood sugar and contribute to weight gain.

A little wine is an
antidote to death; in large
amounts it is the poison of life.

**Persian proverb**

# Chapter 15

# *In Vino Veritas*

Grapes are one of the oldest and most widespread fruits in the world. Fossil analysis indicates that wild vines already existed over 65 million years ago and, aided by climate change, they had spread all over the surface of the globe by 25 million years ago, even to such unexpected places as Alaska and Greenland. However, their distribution became much more restricted during the ice ages that followed, so that by roughly 10,000 years ago wild vines were mainly concentrated around the Caspian Sea, in a region that now corresponds to Georgia and Armenia.

As grapes were very sweet and thus tended to ferment quickly, it is likely that the proximity of human beings and these wild vines rapidly led to the discovery and production of the first fermented drinks made from grapes. No one knows whether the no doubt unusual taste of these first "wines" is what led to later efforts to cultivate vines, but according to the analysis of the oldest seeds from cultivated grapevines found to date, this domestication dates from antiquity (7000–5000 BCE); it appears to have begun in the Caucasus, and then occurred further south in Mesopotamia, where wine-stained amphora dating from 3500 BCE have been found.

This primitive viticulture was later developed considerably by the Egyptians, who believed wine to be a gift from Osiris, god of the dead, its status obvious in the many frescos adorning funeral chambers from Egypt's Third Dynasty (2686–2613 BCE) onward. Its use was restricted to dignitaries in Egypt, and wine production did not spread in any significant way around the Mediterranean until the Greek Empire, when this drink really became a part of broader human culture, an importance symbolized by the cult of Dionysus, the Greek god of wine and drunkenness. Dionysus was replaced by Bacchus after the Roman conquest, and the successors of the Greeks put even more effort into wine growing and trading, not only in Italy but also on the Mediterranean coasts of France and Spain. More than 2,000 years later, these countries remain the main wine exporters worldwide.

## The beneficial effects of wine on health

With the exception of tea, no drink is as inextricably linked with civilization as wine. Interestingly, while its mood-enhancing side has definitely helped make it an essential element of celebrations and festivities, wine has always been thought to be a drink with beneficial health effects. The founder of medicine, Hippocrates, wrote of it that "wine is wonderfully suited to man if, in health as in sickness, it is taken appropriately and in correct amounts, according to the individual constitution." And he did not hesitate to recommend it to treat several diseases. During the Roman Empire, this therapeutic view of wine was still fashionable, and Pliny the Elder (23–79 CE), author of the voluminous *Natural History* we have already mentioned, also thought that "wine in itself is a remedy; it nourishes man's blood, delights the stomach and softens grief and worry." The eruption of Vesuvius in 79 CE prevented Pliny the Elder from continuing to extol wine's virtues, but in spite of everything these beliefs took on greater importance in the Middle Ages, when wine was an integral part of medical practice. The medical treatises of the first medical school in Europe, founded in the 10th century in Salerno, near Naples, Italy, mention that "pure wine has many beneficial effects [...] and gives robust health in life [...] drink some, but make sure it is good."  These recommendations were still in favor a few centuries later at the University of Montpellier (1221), then known as the largest medical school in Europe, where half of the medicinal "recipes" in its books contained wine.

We might think that these ancient beliefs and uses, rooted much more in intuition than in actual medical knowledge, would have disappeared over the following centuries, but on the contrary, far from running out of steam, the role of wine in European medicine just continued to grow until the 19th century. Even Louis Pasteur, who at the time was already extremely famous, considered wine to be "the healthiest and most hygienic of beverages."

It was not until the end of the 20th century that concrete evidence of the ways in which wine can be beneficial to health was gathered. A study of the factors responsible for the mortality associated with heart disease demonstrated that the French, despite a way of life including several known risk factors for cardiovascular diseases (high cholesterol levels, high blood pressure, smoking), have an unusually low mortality associated with these diseases, compared with other countries having the same risk factor levels. For example, in spite of a fat intake similar to that of residents of the United States or the United Kingdom, the French have almost half the number of heart attacks or other coronary events causing premature deaths. As the main difference between the French diet and the Anglo-Saxon diet is the relatively high consumption of wine in France, it was assumed that this "French paradox" could be linked to wine consumption, and especially to red wine consumption.

## Red wine and mortality

Many studies have shown that people who consume moderate amounts of alcohol daily have a lower risk of dying prematurely than those who abstain or who drink too much. The analysis of hundreds of epidemiological studies on the effect of alcohol on mortality in Western populations very clearly shows a response in the form of a "J-curve" with regard to alcohol (Figure 80). Moderate amounts of alcohol (two glasses of about 4 ounces/120

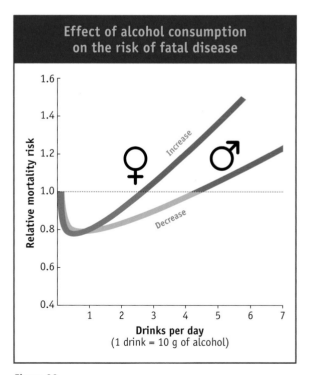

**Figure 80**

ml per day for men and one glass per day for women) significantly decrease the risk of death (by 25 percent to 30 percent), all causes combined. However, if this amount is exceeded, the risk of death increases very rapidly, especially in women.

This positive effect of ethanol seems mainly due to an increase in the blood of HDL, or good cholesterol, considered to be a key factor in protection against heart disease, as well as to a decrease in blood clot formation by inhibiting blood platelet aggregation. Conversely, high doses of alcohol cause considerable cell damage and definitely increase cancer risk — hence the rising arrow for risk of death seen in Figure

80. Alcohol is therefore the perfect example of a double-edged sword that must be used intelligently if we want to make the most of its beneficial effects.

Several studies indicate that the regular and moderate consumption of red wine might offer greater benefits than other kinds of alcohol. For example, moderate red wine drinkers have one-third the risk of dying prematurely than those who prefer beer or spirits (34 percent compared with 10 percent), which suggests that wine's unique phytochemical compound content, especially polyphenols, could have positive effects that greatly exceed those attributable to alcohol. In addition, it is interesting to note that red wine, even dealcoholized, improves blood vessel elasticity, increases the blood's antioxidant capacity and reduces the oxidation of LDL cholesterol, all parameters associated with a decrease in the risk of heart disease. It is therefore likely that the large amounts of phenolic compounds in red wine play an important role in the reduced mortality risk associated with the moderate consumption of this drink.

## Why red wine?

While it may seem surprising for an alcoholic beverage to cause this kind of decrease in the rates of serious diseases like heart disease, it is

| Main phytochemical compounds in wine | | |
|---|---|---|
| Phytochemical compounds | Average concentration (mg/l)* | |
| | Red wine | White wine |
| Anthocyanidins | 281 | 0 |
| Proanthocyanidins | 171 | 7.1 |
| Flavonols | 98 | 0 |
| Phenolic acids | 375 | 210 |
| Resveratrol | 3 | 0.3 |
| **Total** | **1,200** | **217** |

*Given the extreme variability in wine's phytochemical content, the concentrations given are averages of currently available values.

**Figure 81**　　　　Adapted from German and Walzem, 2000.

important to understand that red wine is not just another alcoholic drink. On the contrary, wine is perhaps the most complex drink in the human diet. This complexity stems from the lengthy grape fermentation process, which brings about important changes in the chemical composition of the pulp, making it possible to extract some specific molecules while modifying the structure of several others. The result is impressive, there being several hundred distinct molecules in red wine, notably members of the polyphenol family — 34 ounces (1 l) of red wine can contain up to 2 g of polyphenols (Figure 81).

Since these polyphenols occur mainly in the skins and seeds of grapes, making red wine by fermenting whole grapes means that a much higher amount of compounds is extracted than in making white wine, where the skin and seeds are rapidly removed from the fermentation process.

Among the hundreds of polyphenols in red wine, resveratrol (Figure 82) is the one currently arousing the most interest as the molecule responsible for the beneficial properties associated with moderate red wine consumption. Although this molecule is a relatively minor component of wine in terms of quantity (from 1–7 mg/l compared with 200 mg/l for proanthocyanidins, for example), resveratrol is found exclusively in this drink and could therefore offer a plausible explanation for the beneficial effects of wine.

This interest in resveratrol does not mean, however, that the many other polyphenols plentiful in red wine (anthocyanidins, proanthocyanidins, phenolic acids) make no contribution to the properties of wine; far from it, as we saw in Chapter 11. Still, the results obtained concerning resveratrol's anticancer potential are so dramatic that this molecule has received special attention in recent years.

## Resveratrol

Resveratrol is a plant hormone isolated for the first time in 1940 from the roots of the *Veratrum grandiflorum* plant (resveratrol literally means "the object of veratrum," from *res* "thing" or "object," and *veratrum*),

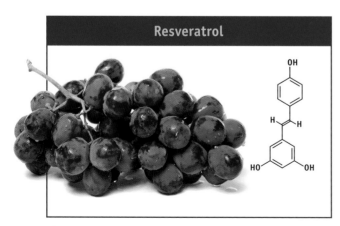

**Resveratrol**

OH

H

H

HO

OH

**Figure 82**

and it was only in 1976 that its presence in grapevines was detected. The production of resveratrol by grapevines is one of the plant's defense mechanisms against environmental stress (thinning out of leaves, for example) or against attacks by microorganisms, like the microscopic fungus *Botrytis cinerea*, which causes noble rot on grapes. In general, grape varieties grown in regions with a more temperate, rainy climate are more likely to be attacked by microorganisms, and as a result have higher resveratrol levels than those grown in less hostile climates. For example, a pinot noir from Burgundy or the Niagara Valley has high concentrations of resveratrol (10 mg/l or more), as the very thin skin of grapes of this variety, as well as their very compact clusters, make them especially vulnerable to attack from microscopic fungi in these humid regions. The resveratrol produced by the plant in reaction to attack by microorganisms is found mostly in the skin and seeds of the fruit, which explains its presence in red wine and its near absence in white wine.

As we have already mentioned, there are relatively few food sources with significant resveratrol content; the best source is without doubt red wine, in which its concentration can be as high as 1 mg per glass of wine (4 ounces/125 ml), depending on the grape variety and the wine's place of origin, of course (Figure 83).

The high amount of resveratrol in red wine can be explained not only by the prolonged fermentation of the must, making possible the extraction of this molecule from the grape seeds and skins, but also by the absence of oxygen in the bottle, which prevents the molecule from oxidizing. This is actually why raisins, while high in polyphenols, do not contain resveratrol, as it is degraded by exposure to air and sunlight.

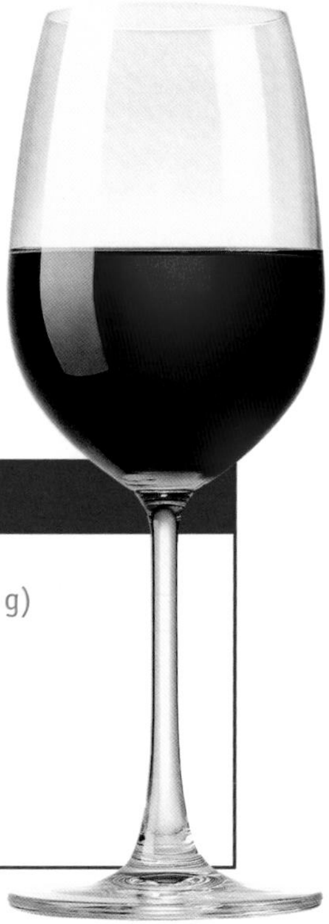

| Resveratrol content in various foods and beverages | | | |
|---|---|---|---|
| Food | Resveratrol (µg/100 g) | Beverage | Resveratrol (µg/100 g) |
| Grapes | 1,500 | Red wine | 625 |
| Peanuts | 150 | White wine | 38 |
| Peanut butter | 50 | Grape juice | 65 |
| Blueberries | 3 | Cranberry juice | 65 |
| Raisins | 0.01 | | |

Figure 83

Resveratrol is obviously also found in large amounts in grapes on the vine, but since it is found in the skin and seeds of the fruit, it is not well absorbed by the body. Peanuts may at first glance appear to be an adequate source of the molecule, but the amount required to reach a high level of resveratrol risks doing more harm than good. Grape juice also contains some, as does cranberry juice, but roughly 10 times less than red wine. This difference can be attributed to the long process of macerating the grape skins during the fermentation into wine that makes the extraction of a large amount of resveratrol from the skins possible. In addition, much more resveratrol is extracted in solutions containing alcohol, which contributes to its increased concentration in red wine. Heat pressing the grapes during the production of grape juice extracts a relatively large amount as well. These juices can thus be a useful source of the molecule, especially for children who, because of their lower blood volume, need a lower intake to reach significant blood concentrations of resveratrol, but also for pregnant women and anyone who does not want to or cannot drink alcohol.

It is also important to note that, despite the lower amount of resveratrol in grape juice, this beverage can be very healthy. Grape juice has very high levels of anthocyanidins, phenolic acids and other polyphenols with a great many chemopreventive and antioxidant properties. Grape juice (as well as red and white wines) also contains high levels of piceid, a resveratrol derivative with glucose in its structure, and it is very possible that the degradation of this glucose by enzymes in the intestinal flora allows large amounts of resveratrol to be released.

Although it is not always clearly established that resveratrol alone is responsible for the beneficial effects of red wine on the incidence of cardiovascular diseases, some evidence does lead us to believe that this molecule plays a major role. Resveratrol has been identified as the active principle in *ko-jo-kon*, a traditional Asian medicine obtained by crushing the roots of the Japanese knotweed, also known as false bamboo (*Polygonum cuspidatum*), which has been used in Asia for thousands of years to treat heart, liver and blood vessel diseases (the resveratrol sold in the West in the form of supplements is often an extract of these roots). Chinese medicine uses the roots of certain varieties of *Veratrum* to treat high blood pressure as well. In India, the Ayurvedic tradition has also for thousands of years used a medicine, darakchasava, made mainly from vine extracts, to enhance cardiac strength. Given the widespread nature of wine in European and Mediterranean cultures, it is somewhat ironic that the first evidence of the beneficial effect of resveratrol on diseases comes once again from the East.

It is interesting to note, however, that cultures in which wine is practically absent have nonetheless managed to identify preparations high in resveratrol for treating heart and circulatory disorders. In our opinion, this example admirably illustrates the concept that we presented earlier, which is that the curiosity and ingenuity of human beings in their search for remedies  to treat their ailments must not be underestimated, and that the detailed analysis of culinary traditions and age-old medicines using modern science can lead to identifying molecules with beneficial health effects.

## Resveratrol's anticancer properties

The negative effects associated with consuming high amounts of alcohol are mainly due to an increase in risk for some types of cancer, especially those of the mouth, larynx, esophagus, colon, liver and breast. These increases in risk are not usually the fault of alcohol per se, but rather of the acetaldehyde produced when it is metabolized. Acetaldehyde is in fact a highly reactive molecule that can cause enormous damage to cells' genetic material, especially in people who smoke as well as drink: heavy drinkers (six glasses or more per day) who smoke more than a pack of

cigarettes daily have up to 40 times more risk of developing cancer of the mouth, larynx or esophagus, owing to the extraordinary increase (700 percent) in the amount of acetaldehyde that comes into contact with the organs.

It seems however that this increased cancer risk is much less pronounced in red wine drinkers and that this beverage might even play a role in preventing some types of cancer. A Danish study showed that the moderate consumption of red wine not only led to a 40 percent reduction in the risk of death linked to heart disease, but also to a reduction in the mortality associated with cancer (22 percent),

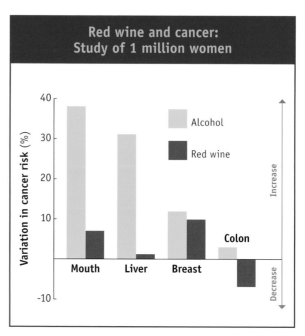

**Figure 84**

with these effects being by far superior to those of moderate consumption of other kinds of alcohol, like beer and spirits. In the same vein, the moderate consumption of red wine is associated with a significant reduction in lung cancer risk, whereas the risk of this cancer increases in beer and spirit drinkers. A reduction in risk for some other cancers (colon, pancreas, esophagus) has also been observed in red wine drinkers, whereas these cancers actually increase in people who drink other kinds of alcoholic beverages. More recently, a study done on a million women clearly showed that while drinking alcohol increases the risk of several types of cancer, this increase is much lower for women who are moderate red wine drinkers. Thus, while just one drink daily of any alcoholic beverage increases the risk of mouth cancer by 38 percent and that of liver cancer by 31 percent, these increases disappear almost completely when consumption is in the form of red wine (Figure 84). Red wine's superiority is also noted in the case of colon cancer, with a decrease in risk of roughly 10 percent, compared with a slight increase associated with moderate alcohol consumption in general. The situation with regard to breast cancer is more complex, however, and it is essential to limit consumption to one glass daily to minimize any increased risk (see p. 235). Nonetheless, the greatest decrease in

mortality associated with the consumption of red wine observed in several studies is likely related not only to a more marked protective effect with regard to heart disease risk, but also to a less harmful effect on cancer risk than other kinds of alcoholic drinks. Red wine really is not a drink like any other!

Although red wine's anticancer potential remains to be clearly established, there is no doubt about the fact that this anticancer activity is in large part due to its resveratrol content. In fact, of all the naturally occurring molecules studied to date that show anticancer activity, resveratrol is unquestionably one of those that arouses the greatest enthusiasm. In 1996, resveratrol was identified as the first molecule of nutritional origin able to interfere with tumor progression because of its ability to inhibit the three stages necessary for cancer development — initiation, promotion and progression (see Chapter 2). It goes without saying that these results have greatly stimulated research into the ways in which resveratrol acts on all of these processes, and it must be said that the results so far are meeting expectations, since resveratrol does indeed have the ability to disrupt several processes essential to tumor development and progression. Just like curcumin, which was discussed in Chapter 9, resveratrol is a very powerful anticancer molecule, whose mode of action compares favorably with several synthetic drugs for limiting the growth of cancer cells.

Studies done to date indicate that resveratrol is well absorbed by the body, which means the molecule enters the bloodstream and can thus act on cells. Although resveratrol is metabolized very quickly and blood concentrations of the original molecule are relatively low, recent data suggest that this does not interfere with its anticancer properties. In fact, one of the molecules produced by modifications in the structure of resveratrol, piceatannol, appears to be even better at causing the death of cancer cells like those of leukemia and melanoma, at blood concentrations that are easily obtainable by absorbing red wine. Furthermore, in preclinical studies where resveratrol has shown its effectiveness in preventing the development of breast, colon and esophageal cancers, the molecule was administered in low doses by mouth, and its concentration in the blood fluctuated from 0.1–2 micromoles per liter, an amount likely to be reached by moderate red wine drinking. We can therefore be optimistic about the effectiveness of resveratrol absorbed through diet.

## Long live resveratrol!

One of the fields of research on resveratrol that is currently causing the most enthusiasm concerns the molecule's ability to increase longevity. It has long been known that reducing calorie intake is the best way to increase the longevity of living organisms. For example, laboratory rats "on a diet" have a 30 percent longer lifespan than their fellow rats who eat as much as they want. This effect appears to be related to the activation of a family of proteins called sirtuins that seem to increase the lifespan of cells by giving them the time needed to repair the DNA damage occurring as part of aging. Even more interesting, from a nutritional point of view, results in recent years indicate that some molecules in the diet, like quercetin and especially resveratrol, are very powerful activators of these proteins and that this activation might increase cell longevity. For example, adding resveratrol to the growth environment of simple single-celled organisms, like yeast, prolongs the cells' lifespan by 80 percent. While normally yeasts live for 19 generations, adding resveratrol increases this lifespan to 34 generations! The trend is the same for more "complex" organisms like worms or fruit flies: resveratrol added to the "diet" of these organisms causes an increase in lifespan of 15 percent for the worms and 29 percent for the flies. Resveratrol thus seems to be able to activate cell repair mechanisms and increase organisms' longevity by mimicking, in a way, the effect of caloric restriction. It is possible, however, that other mechanisms contribute to

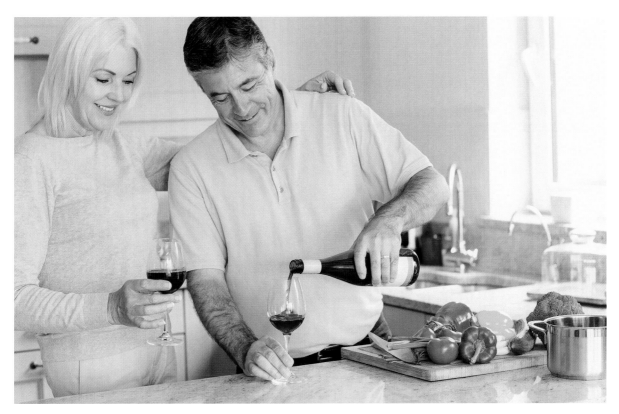

the effect of resveratrol on longevity, since it has recently been discovered that the molecule has the ability to prolong cell life following the activation of several genes whose role is to protect cells, by repairing DNA, for example. This effect of resveratrol is observed in very small doses easily consumed through moderate red wine consumption and might therefore contribute to the increase in life expectancy observed in several organisms after a resveratrol treatment.

Could the decrease in mortality observed in populations who drink red wine moderately be linked to an increase in the lifespan of cells caused by resveratrol? No one can yet say so. One thing is certain, however: given its beneficial effects on the cardiovascular system, and its protection against cancer development, as well as its ability to prolong cell life, resveratrol is likely one of the nutritionally derived molecules with the most beneficial impact on human health.

By including red wine in the list of foods that can contribute to cancer prevention, our intention is not to trivialize the other effects of alcohol consumption — quite the contrary. Drinking too much alcohol, whether or not in the form of red wine, is harmful both in terms of the risk of coronary disease and cancer development, not to mention that it brings in its wake a whole array of serious social problems, ranging from traffic accidents to violent behavior.

Many scientific studies, however, corroborate the range of benefits associated with moderate red wine consumption. Although resveratrol is doubtless not the only factor responsible for all the positive cardiovascular aspects associated with red wine, there is nonetheless little doubt that this molecule is the best source of resveratrol. We must keep in mind that the vast majority of people who drink alcoholic beverages do so in moderation and can, as a result, experience red wine's considerable benefits for preventing chronic diseases like cancer and cardiovascular diseases. Not to mention that red wine drinking is often associated with better quality food,

usually shared in a relaxed atmosphere that reduces the stress that is everywhere in our lives. Remember, however, that countries where red wine consumption has been associated with a lower level of mortality, especially the Mediterranean countries, typically have a diet high in fruits, vegetables, pulses and nuts, use olive oil as a major source of fat and have a moderate meat intake. It is therefore possible, and even highly likely, that the beneficial effects of red wine are greatest when red wine consumption is part of this kind of diet.

In other words, drinking red wine, even moderately, does not guarantee a protective effect against cancer if this consumption is not part of an overall prevention strategy based on a generous intake of other protective foods, like fruits and vegetables, along with a low proportion of bad foods containing large amounts of saturated fat and sweet foods with low nutritional density. In this kind of diet, one or two 4-ounce (125 ml) glasses of wine for men and one for women daily, as recommended by the WCRF, is the amount of wine most likely to prevent cancer and cardiovascular disease from occurring.

**In summary:**

- Red wine is an alcoholic drink unlike any other, containing a great many phytochemical compounds beneficial to health.

- The resveratrol in red wine has a powerful anticancer action that appears to be responsible for the beneficial effects of wine on preventing the development of certain cancers.

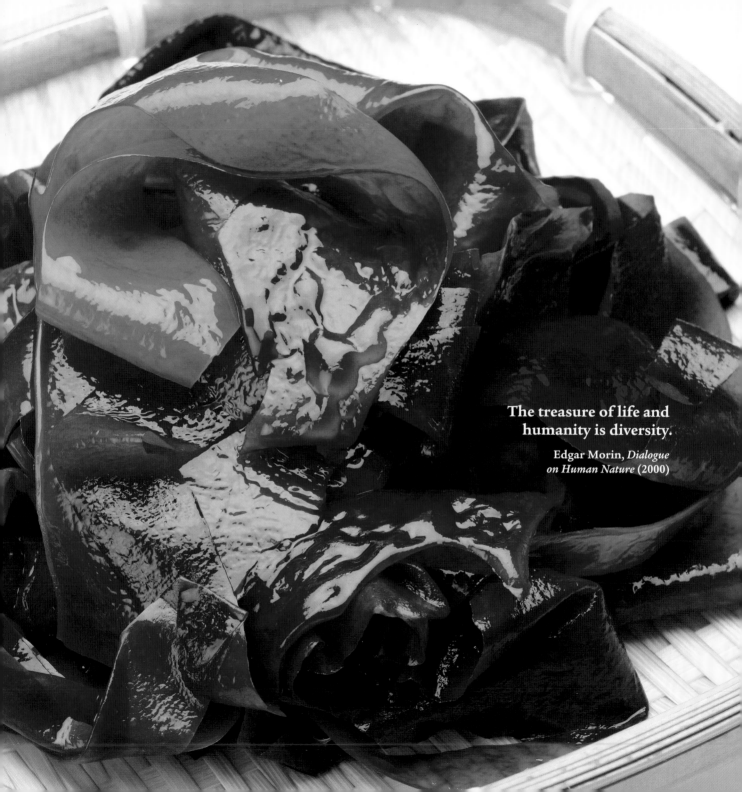

The treasure of life and
humanity is diversity.

Edgar Morin, *Dialogue
on Human Nature* (2000)

# Chapter 16

# Anticancer Biodiversity

All of the organizations dedicated to the prevention of chronic diseases, whether heart disease, diabetes or cancer, agree that eating a minimum of five servings of fruits and vegetables daily is absolutely essential to reduce the incidence and mortality associated with these diseases. Yet, despite this consensus, barely one-quarter of the population follows this recommendation, and fruit and vegetable consumption is actually dropping in some parts of the world. This plant deficiency is especially damaging when it is accompanied by the overconsumption of processed foods, which is often the case. The metabolic imbalances caused by caloric overload promote the creation of an inflammatory environment conducive to the development of chronic diseases; this negative impact is accentuated by the loss of a valuable source of antioxidant and anti-inflammatory molecules resulting from the lack of plants in the diet. There can be no doubt that increased consumption of all fruits and vegetables is an essential prerequisite for any approach to preventing chronic diseases, cancer included.

While the foods discussed in the preceding chapters have outstanding anticancer properties and must as a result be given priority in the daily diet so as to prevent cancer, this does not mean they are the only plants with positive effects. Research in recent years has identified several phytochemical compounds with the potential to interfere in the processes involved in cancer development in varying degrees, and eating foods containing these molecules really can help reduce cancer risk.

## Fiber, to nourish the 100,000 billion bacteria living inside us

Dietary fiber is unquestionably the best example of the importance of increasing our total consumption of plants to prevent cancer. This fiber, mainly found in legumes, cereal grains (whole grains), nuts, fruits and vegetables, consists of complex carbohydrates that resist digestion by the enzymes in the human body and are therefore not absorbed by the intestines. While this lack of nutritional value may at first seem disadvantageous, fiber is on the contrary absolutely essential for maintaining good health and is even among the first components in food to have been associated with lower cancer risk.

Fiber's anticancer potential was first suggested in 1971 by British scientist David Burkitt, following his observation that the inhabitants of rural parts of Africa, who ate large amounts of fiber, had an abnormally low incidence of colon cancer, several times lower than that of Westerners, who ate very little fiber. The protective effect of dietary fiber has been confirmed by numerous studies, and recent analyses indicate that every 0.35 ounces (10 g) of fiber in food is associated with a reduction of roughly 15 percent in colorectal cancer risk. This positive effect does not however seem to be limited to intestinal cancers, since the regular consumption of dietary fiber has also been associated with a decrease in liver and breast cancer risk (Figure 85).

The beneficial impact of dietary fiber on cancer risk is in large part a result of its transformation by intestinal bacteria. This huge bacterial community, called the microbiome, can itself be considered an organ, both because of the astronomical number of cells it contains

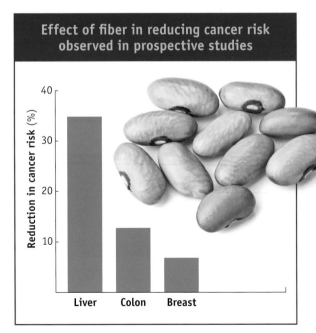

**Effect of fiber in reducing cancer risk observed in prospective studies**

Reduction in cancer risk (%)

Liver    Colon    Breast

**Figure 85**

214

(100,000 billion bacteria, or 10 times the number of cells in the whole human body) and because of its activities, which are absolutely essential to our body's harmonious functioning. The breaking down of plant fiber by the fermentation activity of these intestinal bacteria results in the production of several short-chain fatty acids (butyrate, acetate, propionate) which have a powerful anti-inflammatory effect on the immune system and therefore an anticancer action. At the same time, the fermentation of fiber creates lactic acid, slightly acidifying the intestine and thus slowing down the proliferation of many pathogenic microorganisms, which prefer more hospitable conditions in which to grow; this reduces inflammation and the production of certain carcinogenic compounds. In short, regular fiber consumption results in a diversified microbiome, composed mainly of beneficial bacteria that create an anti-inflammatory environment resistant to cancer development.

Several observations suggest that an imbalance in microbiome composition is associated with an increase in cancer risk. For example, the study of intestinal bacteria in patients with colon cancer shows a decrease in bacteria that produce anti-inflammatory fatty acids (butyrate), while the bacteria whose metabolism produces inflammatory molecules are significantly increased. Colorectal adenomas and carcinomas also contain high levels of

certain pathogenic bacteria (*Fusobacterium* spp.) that produce an inflammatory micro-environment conducive to cancer progression. These differences could also contribute to the onset of liver cancer in overweight people, since these individuals are home to larger amounts of bacteria that produce desoxycholic acid, a bile derivative that attacks the DNA in hepatocytes and causes genetic mutations. Lastly, we should mention that a huge number of recent studies also show that a disruption of this bacterial community is associated with numerous metabolic (obesity, diabetes), immunological (allergies) and even neurological (anxiety, autism) problems, which shows just how crucial our relationship with the microbiome is to maintaining good health.

The Western diet is very low in fiber (0.5 ounces/15 g per day instead of the 1–1.5 ounces/30–40 g recommended), and there is no doubt that this deficiency contributes to the high incidence of colorectal cancer in our society. Furthermore, studies show that after just two weeks on a Western diet, high in fat, meat and simple sugars, but low in fiber, a change in the microbiome and an increase in inflammation are already seen in the colon, two advance warning signs for cancer. It also seems that sweeteners (aspartame, sucralose) and some emulsifiers (polysorbate 80), two classes of ingredients widely used in the food industry and occurring everywhere in our food, disrupt the balance of the microbiome and also lead to the development of inflammatory conditions. The almost total absence of fiber, combined with the negative impact of these synthetic molecules, thus creates optimal conditions for the progression of colorectal cancer.

All the same, there is reason to be optimistic: these changes in the bacterial flora are not irreversible, and simply incorporating an abundance of plants, especially those high in fiber (Figure 86), into dietary habits quickly reestablishes the levels of good bacteria and decreases inflammation. We should however be wary of processed products enriched with fiber:

| Examples of high-fiber foods | | | |
|---|---|---|---|
| | Food | Serving | Fiber content (g) |
| Legumes | Lentils | 1 cup | 15.6 |
| | Black beans | 1 cup | 15 |
| Fruits and vegetables | Artichoke | 1 (medium) | 10.3 |
| | Green peas | 1 cup | 8.8 |
| | Raspberries | 1 cup | 8.0 |
| | Broccoli | 1 cup | 5.5 |
| | Pears (with skin) | 1 (medium) | 5.5 |
| Grains and pasta | Whole wheat spaghetti | 1 cup | 6.3 |
| | Bran cereals | ¾ cup | 5.3 |
| | Whole wheat or multigrain bread | 1 slice | 1.9 |
| Nuts and seeds | Sunflower seeds | ¼ cup | 3.9 |
| | Almonds | 1 oz. (23 almonds) | 3.5 |
| | Pistachios | 1 oz. (49 pistachios) | 2.9 |

**Figure 86**

Adapted from the USDA National Nutrient Database for Standard Reference, 2012.

these foods usually contain just one kind of fiber and can in no way match the diversity and complexity of the soluble and insoluble dietary fiber naturally found in plants and absolutely essential to establishing a balanced microbiome.

## Mushroom magic

Mushrooms are an extremely diverse living kingdom, composed of roughly 100,000 species, of which at least 2,000 are edible and 500 are recognized as having, in various degrees, an influence on the functions of the human body. The current body of knowledge about the nutritional, toxic or hallucinogenic properties of mushrooms is the result of much trial and error on the part of human beings, for whom the abundance of these plants in their environment must have been a major source of nutrition. In fact, mushrooms have always held a special place in most of the great culinary traditions, often even attaining the status of a "superior" food, a synonym for luxury and refinement, and therefore especially prized by the wealthy and powerful. Fortunately, eating these delicious mushrooms is no longer the exclusive right of kings, and the domestication of several species has helped make them available year round. Whether we choose button mushrooms or their cremini and Portobello cousins, oyster

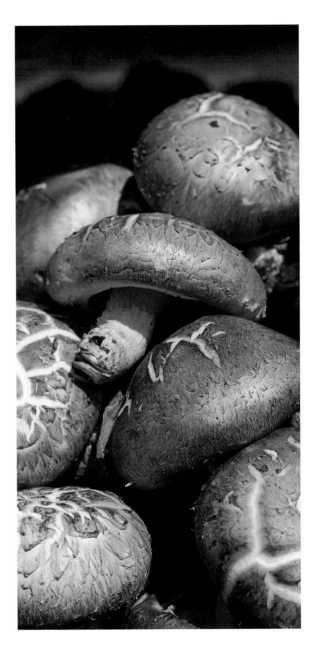

mushrooms, or the various Asian mushrooms (shiitake, enokitake, maitake and shimeji), we have the good fortune to be able to enjoy these delicious foods and their many fine qualities daily, both for their nutritional value and to prevent chronic diseases.

### The anticancer properties of mushrooms

In addition to their culinary properties, mushrooms have always been an important component of traditional medicines in many countries, especially in Asia. With regard to preventing cancer, the results of epidemiological studies that have examined the relationship between eating mushrooms and a reduction in the risk of developing cancer are encouraging. For example, research done in Japan (Nagano Prefecture) highlighted the fact that farmers whose main occupation was cultivating enokitake (and who ate them regularly) had a cancer-related mortality rate 40 percent below that of the population in general. Another study in Japan showed that the regular consumption of *Hypsizygus marmoreus* (shimeji) and *Pholiota nameko* (nameko), two mushrooms popular in the country, was associated with a decrease of approximately 50 percent in stomach cancer risk, with these preventive effects also being observed in laboratory animals treated with a powerful carcinogenic substance, methylcholanthene. In the same vein, an analysis of several studies done on the impact of mushrooms on breast cancer has shown that eating 0.35 ounces (10 g) of mushrooms daily is associated with a risk reduction of about 20 percent. In line with these results, we have recently observed that adding mushroom extracts to cancer cells isolated from a mammary tumor halted the growth of these cells, with the inhibiting effect especially dramatic for enokitake and oyster mushrooms.

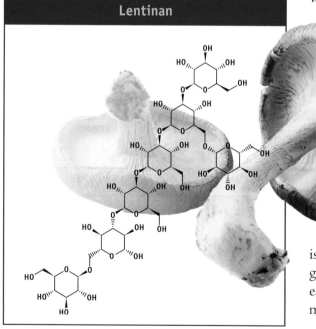

**Lentinan**

**Figure 87**

Several studies indicate that a large number of polysaccharides, complex polymers made up of many units of certain sugars, are responsible for the anticancer effects associated with several mushrooms. These polymers, of varying composition and structure, are found in large amounts in many Asian mushrooms, especially shiitake, enokitake and maitake.

Lentinan (Figure 87), a compound found in shiitake, is a polysaccharide whose antitumor activity is relatively well documented. In patients with stomach or colon cancer, adding lentinan to chemotherapy causes a significant regression in tumors and prolongs survival when compared with chemotherapy alone, suggesting that this polysaccharide has anticancer activity. Furthermore, the administration of a polysaccharide preparation similar to lentinan, PSK, is currently used in Japan in combination with chemotherapy to treat several types of cancer, especially those of the stomach, colon and lung; adding this extract to cytotoxic treatments improves survival rates for patients in remission.

The mechanisms responsible for the anticancer action of the polysaccharides in mushrooms are very complex, but it is now agreed that these compounds stimulate the activity of the immune system. For example, many studies have shown that the lentinan in shiitake and a polysaccharide isolated from maitake both cause a major increase in the number of white blood cells and in the activity of these key cells in the immune system, thus enhancing the effectiveness of the chemotherapy. It seems therefore that the stimulation of immune system activity by the active compounds in these mushrooms increases the chances of being able to control emerging tumors and prevent them from reaching a mature stage.

The anticancer and immunostimulant activity of edible mushrooms is not restricted to Asian species. Oyster and button mushrooms, for example, also contain molecules that seem to be effective in slowing down the development of some cancers, notably colon cancer, by directly attacking the cancer cells and forcing them to die by apoptosis. Similarly, button mushrooms also contain molecules able to prevent the growth of some cancer cells, especially breast cancer cells. This property is attributable to mushrooms' ability to block the action of aromatase, an enzyme that plays a key role in the production of estrogens, the female sex hormones. Since most breast cancers are hormone dependent — that is to say, their progression depends on these estrogens — blocking aromatase causes a drop in estrogen levels and may thus prevent these cancers from progressing. Furthermore, it is interesting to note that administering button mushroom extracts to laboratory animals with breast tumors causes a pronounced regression of these tumors. A protective effect of button mushrooms has also been observed for ovarian cancer, with a reduction of 32 percent in women who eat more than 2 g of these mushrooms a day. As for Asian mushrooms, these positive effects may be linked to an improved immune response, as studies show that administering extracts of these mushrooms leads to a decrease in immunosuppressant factors.

In conclusion, studies done on the anticancer properties of mushrooms have mainly focused on the use of polysaccharides isolated from these plants as immunomodulators designed to improve the effectiveness of chemotherapy and the overall well-being of patients. The positive results obtained are extremely encouraging, especially if we consider the severity of some cases and the difficulty of treating them. In light of these results, there is no doubt that mushrooms can play an important role in cancer prevention, by positively stimulating the immune system so as to enhance the effectiveness of the response to attack from a cancer cell trying to grow.

## Algae — cancer yields to their siren song

Algae appeared on Earth about 1.5 billion years ago and are the ancestors of today's land plants.

Algae were actually the first living species able to convert the sun's energy into substances necessary for cell function through the process of photosynthesis; this was an innovation that benefited them enormously, for there are now no fewer than 10,000 species of algae spread all over the planet's seashores.

In addition to their essential role in the planet's ecology, algae are the prototype of the ideal healthy food. They are very rich in essential minerals (iodine, potassium, iron, calcium), proteins, essential amino acids (all of them), vitamins and fiber. In addition, their fats are in large part the essential fatty acids omega-3 and omega-6, in an ideal ratio of 1:1, and some algae, like nori, even contain long-chain omega-3 fatty acids, like those in fatty fish. The nutritional value of algae, these "sea vegetables," puts them in a class apart, and they deserve a place of honor in the diet. Nori, kombu, wakamé, aramé or dulse are all truly exceptional foods, both nutritionally and gastronomically speaking.

*The anticancer properties of algae*
As we mentioned earlier, the enormous differences in the rates of several cancers between inhabitants of Asian and Western countries are largely related to major differences in the nature of the diets of these populations. Algae definitely represent one of the most striking differences: almost

unknown in the West (with the exception of the Scots and Irish), algae may make up as much as 10 percent of the daily diet of the Japanese, which amounts to nearly 4.4 pounds (2 kg) of algae per person per year! It is not surprising therefore that the Japanese are among the only human beings to have in their intestinal flora a bacteria that has acquired, in the course of evolution, the enzymes porphyranase and agarase, which facilitate the digestion of the polysaccharides in the algae, notably nori, nature's gift to sushi fans!

Japanese women have one of the lowest rates of breast cancer in the world, and several studies have suggested that this protection could be linked to longer menstrual cycles as well as to blood estrogen levels lower than in Western women, two factors that decrease the exposure of tissues targeted by these hormones (breast, endometrium and ovaries) and, as a result, the risk of developing cancer. Recent studies indicate that, in addition to soy phytoestrogens, marine algae might also play a role. The consumption of algae by laboratory animals causes a 37 percent increase in the length of the menstrual cycle as well as a significant decline in blood estrogen levels. These results are certainly representative of the

effect of algae on humans, as a study done on premenopausal women produced similar results, with a significant increase in the length of the menstrual cycle and a decrease in blood estrogens. Algae might therefore be important foods for preventing hormone-dependent cancers, and their antiestrogenic action likely contributes to the low incidence of these cancers in populations that consume large amounts of algae. For example, it is interesting to note that one study recently observed that Korean women who ate the most nori algae had 56 percent less risk of getting breast cancer. Protection against colorectal cancer has also been observed in some studies, suggesting that algae could be multipurpose anticancer foods, active against several types of tumors.

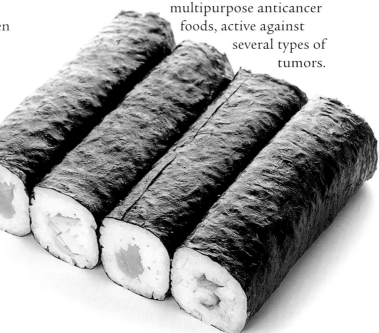

According to recent studies, algae can also interfere with the development of cancer by acting directly on cancer cells. In fact, adding algae extracts to the diet of laboratory animals significantly reduces the cancer development caused by carcinogenic substances, including breast, colon and skin cancers. Even though the mechanisms responsible for these anticancer properties are still poorly understood, there is no doubt they are largely linked to algae's high fucoxanthin and fucoidan content (from the Greek *phukos*, "algae"), two compounds that interfere with several processes essential for the growth of cancer cells.

Fucoidan, a complex sugar polymer plentiful in some algae, especially kombu and wakamé, prevents the growth of a wide variety of cancer cells and even causes these cells to die by apoptosis. In addition to its cytotoxic activity, fucoidan also seems to have a positive impact on immune function by increasing the activity of cells involved in defending against pathogenic agents, which may help create an environment more hostile to microtumors and restrict their development.

Fucoxanthin (Figure 88) is a yellow pigment that, depending on its concentration, gives plants a color ranging from olive green to reddish brown. A close relative of other pigments in the carotenoid family (beta-carotene, lycopene, etc.), fucoxanthin occurs widely in nature, but mainly in sea plants, where it participates in photosynthesis due to its unique ability to absorb sunlight in deep water. Of all the dietary carotenoids tested to date, fucoxanthin is one of those that shows the greatest anticancer activity, both in laboratory animals and on cells isolated from human tumors. For example, adding fucoxanthin to cells taken from a prostate

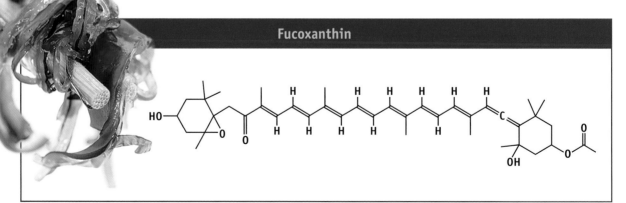

**Figure 88**

cancer causes a significant decrease in the growth of these cells; this inhibiting effect is even much greater than that of lycopene, a carotenoid found mainly in tomatoes and that has long been touted as playing a preventive role in the development of prostate cancer. Since algae are the only food source of fucoxanthin, they should be part of any dietary cancer-prevention strategy, especially with regard to breast and prostate cancer.

In conclusion, marine algae must be considered not just as culinary curiosities, but as actual cancer-preventing foods, able to counteract the progression of latent microtumors both by acting directly on their growth and by positively influencing the immune system and inflammatory processes.

## Pomegranates, new weapons in the fight against cancer!

Native to the Middle East (Iran, Turkey, south of the Caspian Sea), where they were already being cultivated 6,000 years ago, pomegranates have long been considered by the region's inhabitants to be an exceptional fruit, both because of their appearance and unique taste and for their many medicinal properties.

The pomegranate is indeed a very unusual fruit (a large berry, in fact) containing several hundred arils, seeds consisting of a translucent red pulp with a sweet and sour taste. These arils are a genuine "explosion" of antioxidants owing to their exceptional levels of two large groups of polyphenols: anthocyanins, which give the pomegranate its characteristic red color, and hydrolyzable tannins, like punicalin, punicalagin and other derivatives of ellagic acid.

Data accumulated to date indicate that this remarkable polyphenol content gives pomegranates powerful anticancer activity, as these molecules have the ability to inhibit the growth of cells from colon, breast, lung and prostate cancers. In the latter case, preclinical studies show that giving pomegranate juice to animals with prostatic tumors leads to a substantial reduction in the growth of these tumors, as well as a decrease in PSA levels, a marker for cancer progression. This protective effect is also observed in clinical studies done on patients with prostate cancer who have undergone surgery or radiotherapy; whereas PSA levels in these patients usually double 15 months after treatment, reflecting the rapid growth of residual cancer cells, this progression is nearly four times slower (54 months) in those who consume 8 ounces (250 ml) of pomegranate juice daily. Interestingly, a clinical trial recently showed that an extract containing pomegranate in combination with turmeric, green tea and broccoli caused a dramatic reduction in PSA levels in prostate cancer patients. The positive effect of pomegranates on the evolution of clinically confirmed prostate cancer even at an advanced stage indicates that this fruit possesses enormous preventive potential to slow down the progression of this disease at earlier stages, when the cancer cells have not yet reached their full strength. In this regard, it must be noted that regions where pomegranates have been part of the diet for thousands of years, for example in countries around the Caspian Sea (Uzbekistan, Turkmenistan, Azerbaijan), have the lowest incidence of prostate cancer in the world, almost 50 times lower than in the West.

| Chlorogenic acid content of fruits in the *Rosaceae* Family | |
| --- | --- |
| Fruit | Chlorogenic acids content (mg/100 g) |
| Apples | 119 |
| Pears | 59 |
| Plums | 44 |
| Nectarines | 28 |
| Peaches | 24 |
| Apricots | 17 |
| Cherries | 12 |

The values represent the highest amounts measured in certain varieties.

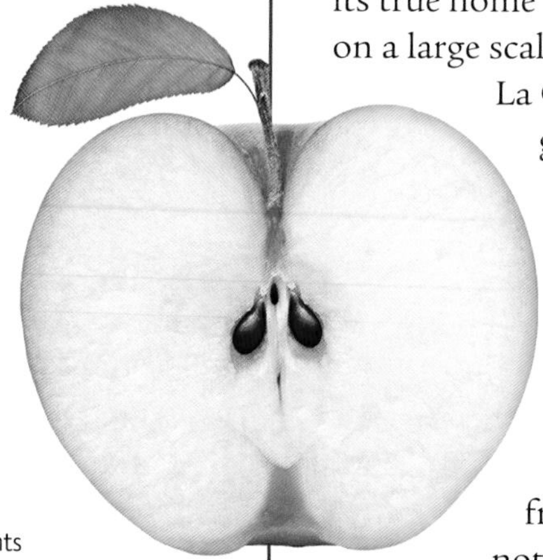

**Figure 89**     Adapted from C. Andres-Lacueva et al., 2009.

## Peaches, a cancer-fighting guilty pleasure

The peach tree (*Prunus persica*) is native to the Tarim Basin, in northwestern China, where it was domesticated and cultivated about 4,000 years ago. A symbol of long life and immortality, the peach has always occupied a place of honor in Chinese culture, as attested to by its pervasiveness in fables and works of art, and as decoration on gifts to loved ones. This love for peaches is obviously not limited to China, and the cultivation of the fruit rapidly spread to the West, first to Persia, following its conquest by Alexander the Great (hence its botanical name of *persica*), and then Europe. Not especially popular with the Romans, who preferred apricots (for Pliny, peaches were a fruit without perfume and of little interest), the peach found its true home in France, where it was cultivated on a large scale beginning in the 15th century. La Quintanie, Louis the XIV's gardener, actually succeeded in cultivating about 30 different species (including the famous Téton de Vénus) to satisfy the Sun King's passion for peaches. Although most of these peach varieties were the result of manipulations carried out by the fruit growers of the day, it must be noted that the nectarine is a natural peach variety that appeared following the spontaneous mutation of the gene responsible for the fruit's fuzzy skin.

### The anticancer properties of peaches

Peaches, like their close relatives in the *Prunus* genus (plums, apricots, cherries, almonds) and several other fruits like apples and pears, belong to the botanical family called *Rosaceae*. Although they look and taste very different, the fruits in this family have the common trait of containing significant amounts of hydroxycinnamic acids, especially chlorogenic and neochlorogenic acids (Figure 89), and this class of polyphenols likely contributes to the anticancer properties of these foods.

This anticancer potential was highlighted in a study done on 47,000 women showing that apple and pear consumption was associated with a reduction of roughly 30 percent in lung cancer risk. Similarly, an analysis of the food habits of 490,802 Americans shows that high consumption of peaches, nectarines, pears and apples is associated with a 40 percent decrease in risk for head and neck cancer.

The anticancer effects specifically associated with eating peaches have been little studied, but preliminary results are very promising. For example, peach extracts containing chlorogenic and neochlorogenic acids are able to specifically block the growth of breast cancer cells, whereas they have no effect at all on normal noncancerous cells. In preclinical models, this inhibiting effect is reflected in a major reduction in tumor growth and the formation of metastases, at polyphenol levels that can easily be reached through diet (two peaches). These observations are consistent with recent studies showing that regular consumption of peaches and nectarines is associated with a significant decrease (40 percent) in some types of breast cancer (Figure 38, p. 80). Given the current state of knowledge, there is therefore no doubt that peaches and nectarines are very valuable additions to the diet of everyone who wants to lower their risk of breast cancer.

## A little coffee to prevent cancer?

Legend has it that a shepherd in Abyssinia (now Ethiopia) discovered the coffee bush when he noticed that his goats were livelier after eating berries from this bush, which grows wild in the region. While this story is impossible to verify, coffee's stimulating properties are not in doubt: caffeine is a very active alkaloid that quickly reaches the brain, where it causes the levels of dopamine to rise and stimulates nerve activity. Drinking coffee thus temporarily increases alertness, a stimulant effect that seems to be especially prized by humans, since every year roughly 132,000 tons (120,000 tonnes) of caffeine are consumed worldwide, making it the most popular psychoactive substance in the world.

In addition to their caffeine content, coffee beans contain no fewer than 800 different phytochemical compounds that might have a beneficial influence on the human body. Among these, we should mention the diterpenes cafestol and kahweal, which speed up the elimination of carcinogenic substances, cafeic and chlorogenic acids, which have strong antioxidant activity, and

a wide array of other polyphenols with well-documented positive effects. Much more than just a stimulant, coffee is therefore a highly complex beverage, containing a wide range of phytochemical molecules performing many biological activities.

### Coffee's anticancer properties

Currently available data indicate that regular coffee consumption is associated with a reduction in risk for some types of cancer. The analysis of roughly 60 population studies indicates that regular coffee drinkers have approximately a 20 percent lower risk of getting cancer than people who never or very seldom drink it. This protective effect is observed for several types of cancer (bladder, mouth, colon, esophagus, uterus, brain and skin), but is especially well documented for liver cancer: people who regularly drink coffee have roughly 40 percent less risk of getting this disease (Figure 90). Another study reported that women who drink substantial amounts of coffee (five or more cups a day) see their risk of getting breast cancer decrease by 20 percent compared with those who drink only one cup or less per day. The protective impact of coffee is especially dramatic for a subtype of breast cancer called ER- (which does not involve estrogen receptors), with a 57 percent reduction in risk among coffee drinkers. This result is interesting, since

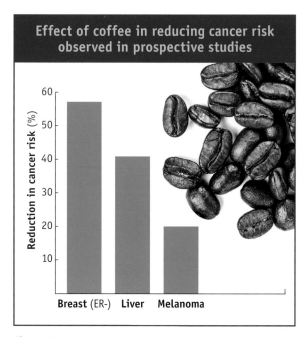

**Figure 90**    Adapted from C. Andres-Lacueva et al., 2009.

ER- tumors make up about one-third of breast cancers and are responsible for many deaths, owing to their resistance to current treatments. Coffee might thus significantly reduce recurrences in women who have fought hormone-dependent breast cancer and are being treated with tamoxifen, since moderate coffee consumption is associated with a 50 percent reduction in recurrence.

Caffeine's stimulant effect can be enjoyed through moderate coffee consumption (two or three cups a day); this is a good way to satisfy cravings for this mild drug, while making the most of the enormous potential of molecules in plant-based foods. On the other hand, energy drinks high in caffeine are not a good alternative, first because they are totally empty from a nutritional point of view, and second because they cause many side effects when consumed in excessive amounts.

## Chocolate, food of the gods

The cacao tree appears to have been domesticated at least 3,000 years ago in the Yucatan region of Mexico. The Mayans, as well as their successors, the Toltecs and especially the Aztecs, attached great importance to the beans of this tree, which they used as currency, as well as to make a bitter, spicy drink called *xocoatl*. When conquistador Hernán Cortés landed on the Mexican coast in April 1519, the Aztec emperor of the day, Montezuma II, welcomed him as a god by offering him gold, plantations and … a chocolate drink in a goblet encrusted with gold. Cortés was, however, much more attracted by the treasures of the Aztec civilization than by chocolate and made the most of the situation to conquer Tenochtitlan (Mexico), the capital of the Empire. This was the end of the Aztec civilization, but the beginning of chocolate's

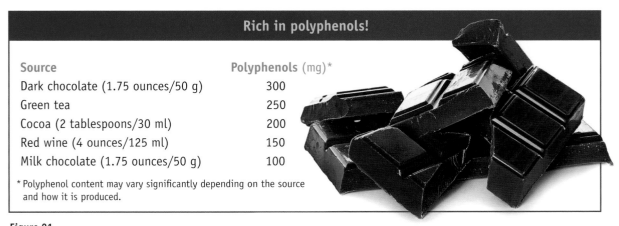

| Rich in polyphenols! | |
|---|---|
| **Source** | **Polyphenols** (mg)* |
| Dark chocolate (1.75 ounces/50 g) | 300 |
| Green tea | 250 |
| Cocoa (2 tablespoons/30 ml) | 200 |
| Red wine (4 ounces/125 ml) | 150 |
| Milk chocolate (1.75 ounces/50 g) | 100 |

\* Polyphenol content may vary significantly depending on the source and how it is produced.

**Figure 91**

invasion of the world, for immediately on its arrival in Europe, chocolate quickly established itself as a food with a divine taste, a unique power to attract and the ability to arouse gluttony and passion. In 1753, when Linnaeus the botanist suggested naming the cacao bush *Theobroma cacao*, which literally means "food of the gods," there was no objection!

### The beneficial effects of dark chocolate

Interest in the beneficial effects of dark chocolate comes from its high phytochemical compound content: a single square of dark chocolate contains twice as many polyphenols as a glass of red wine and as many as a cup of green tea steeped for a long time (Figure 91). The main polyphenols in cacao are the same as those found in large amounts in green tea (catechins); the polymers formed from these molecules, proanthocyanidins (see p. 167), can make up between 12 percent and 48 percent of the weight of the cacao bean. Given the many biological activities associated with these molecules, it is therefore likely that chocolate may have beneficial effects on health.

Dark chocolate's positive impact on cardiovascular diseases is especially well documented. Population studies in fact indicate that the regular consumption of 0.18–0.35 ounces (5–10 g) of 70 percent dark chocolate is associated with a significant decrease in mortality related to these diseases (50 percent), apparently owing to the many beneficial effects of the polyphenols in cacao on the cardiovascular system: an increase in nitrous oxide production, a molecule that stimulates arterial dilation and lowers blood pressure; a reduction in the formation of blood clots by decreasing platelet aggregation and blood levels of certain inflammatory molecules (C-reactive protein); and an increase in the blood's antioxidant capacity, which decreases the oxidation of proteins responsible for the formation of atheromatous plaques. It is interesting to note that these cardiovascular effects cause better circulation of blood to the brain, which could contribute to the significant improvement in memory and cognitive functions observed following chocolate consumption. As emphasized in an article published in the prestigious *New England Journal of Medicine*, it is not surprising that populations who eat the most chocolate are also those that have the highest number of Nobel Prize winners!

The high amounts of polyphenols in dark chocolate also make it possible to foresee a positive role for this food in cancer prevention. It has been known for several years that people who eat the largest amounts of flavonoids have a lower risk of getting several types of cancer, especially bladder, ovarian, prostate, liver and lung cancer. Although the contribution of the flavonoids in chocolate to these protective effects has not been specifically studied, there is every reason to be optimistic. For example, it has been observed that eating 1.6 ounces (45 g) of dark chocolate containing 860 mg of polyphenols was associated with a pronounced decrease in DNA damage in blood cells caused by oxidative stress, which lowers the risk of mutations that can trigger cancer. These results concur with several preclinical studies showing that the polyphenols in cocoa paste have strong anticancer and antiangiogenic activity and are able to slow down the development of several types of cancer in laboratory animals, colon cancer in particular. In the latter case, this protective effect may be linked to a reduction in inflammation, as the majority of polyphenols reach the colon, where they are changed by the intestinal bacteria into phenolic acids and into short-chain fatty acids with anti-inflammatory properties. Just as with fruits and vegetables, including dark chocolate in our eating habits could therefore have important benefits for the proper functioning of the intestine and, by extension, for the prevention of colorectal cancer.

The daily consumption of 0.7 ounces (20 g) of dark chocolate containing 70 percent cocoa can supply the body with a very valuable ration of polyphenols and, as a result, provide benefits in terms of preventing cardiovascular diseases and cancer. This preventive effect will be even greater if eating dark chocolate helps reduce intake of sugary foods and other sweets that contain no anticancer compounds and lead to excess weight. In other words, while we accept that sugar consumption is now part of our eating habits because of the feeling of well-being it gives us, changing these habits by substituting dark chocolate for commonly eaten sugary foods can have a significant impact on the prevention of chronic diseases like cancer. Who said that eating a healthy diet had to be unpleasant?

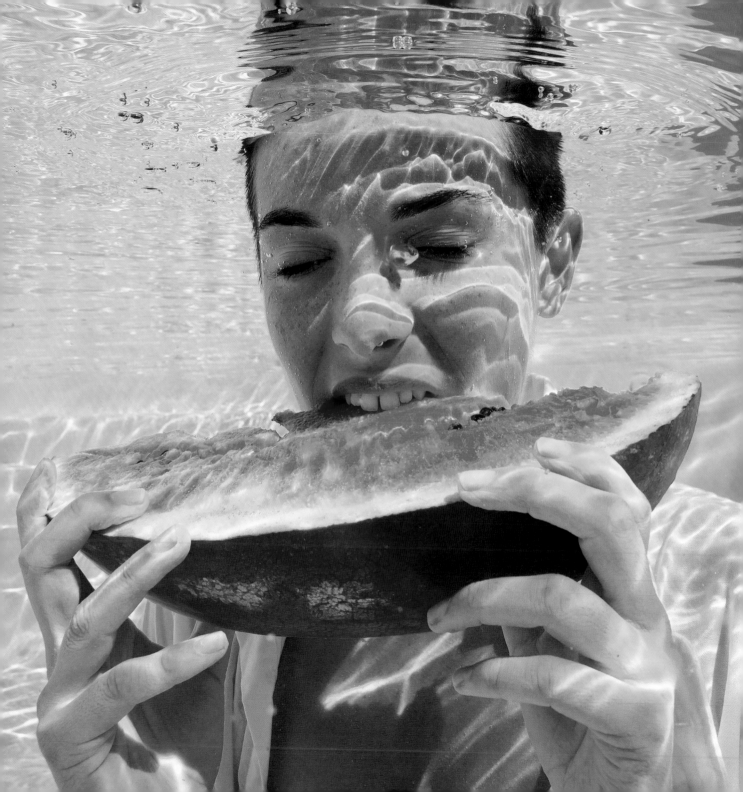

# Part III:

# Day-to-day cancer prevention

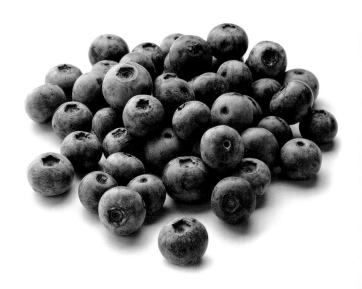

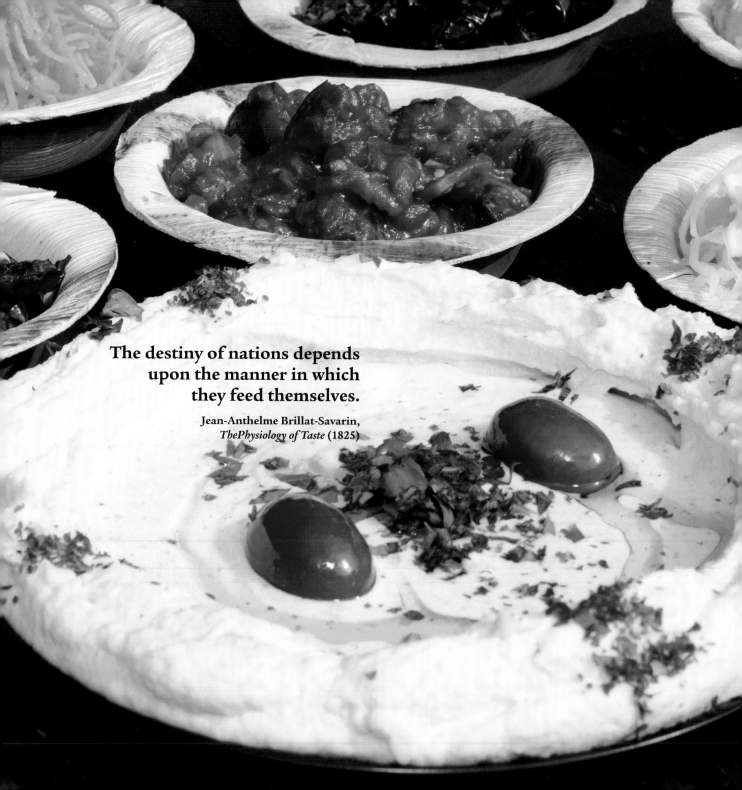

The destiny of nations depends
upon the manner in which
they feed themselves.

Jean-Anthelme Brillat-Savarin,
*ThePhysiology of Taste* (1825)

# Chapter 17

# On the Menu: Fighting Cancer!

The main characteristic of the Western diet is its extremist approach — both its excesses and its shortcomings: too much sugar, too much fat and too much red meat on the one hand; not enough fruits, vegetables and dietary fiber on the other. Reestablishing balance in the dietary intake of these two extremes while avoiding poor-quality foods as much as possible (junk food especially) can only have beneficial consequences for preventing chronic diseases like cancer. Inspired by the recommendations of various cancer-fighting bodies like the World Cancer Research Fund, the American Cancer Society and the Canadian Cancer Society, it is possible to come up with nine broad principles that can have an enormous impact on the risk of getting cancer.

## 1. Stop smoking

Since one-third of cancers are directly caused by smoking, it goes without saying that quitting smoking is one of the changes in habit that can have the greatest impact on cancer prevention. The list of harmful effects associated with tobacco is a long one: a 40 times higher risk of getting lung cancer, a significant increase in cancers of the aerodigestive system (mouth, larynx), pancreas and bladder, a striking increase in risk for fatal cardiovascular diseases, not to mention the various unpleasant side effects associated with tobacco use, like the loss of the senses of smell and taste, chronic fatigue, etc.

Fortunately, our societies have made giant strides in controlling smoking; intensive information campaigns on the dangers of tobacco, more and more widespread bans on smoking in public places and increases in the price of tobacco products have all had the direct result of significantly reducing the proportion of smokers in our societies. Today, even the most seasoned smokers admit that smoking is harmful to health, and most of them express the desire to change their habits. These people should not feel any shame or embarrassment if they have trouble quitting smoking: nicotine is one of the most powerful drugs found in nature and it creates a dependency that is extremely hard to fight. We can only encourage smokers who want to quit smoking to use every means currently at their disposal (electronic cigarettes, nicotine patches, pharmacological products) to help them end their dependency. Quitting smoking is by far the decision that will have the most impact on the quality of your life.

## 2. Get enough exercise

Exercise is not just a good habit for maintaining flexibility and muscle tone: many studies show unequivocally that regular physical activity significantly reduces the risk for several cancers, especially colon and breast cancer. Being physically active does not just mean using your muscles; it also causes a series of biochemical and physiological changes that reduce chronic inflammation inside the body, thus depriving still immature cancer cells of a tool indispensable for their growth. Not to mention that regular physical activity helps maintain a normal body weight, an essential part of cancer prevention. Numerous studies show that a sedentary way of life is associated with a significant increase in cancer risk, especially for colon, breast, lung and uterine cancer.

Regular physical activity is especially important for people who have had cancer. Many studies have in fact shown that cancer survivors who are the most physically active are also those who live the longest, an especially well-documented effect for breast and colon cancer. You do not have to start an Olympic fitness program to get the most out of exercise: in every study, regular fast walking, for example from three to five hours a week, was the activity most commonly associated with a decrease in cancer risk or recurrence. The most important thing is to realize that being sedentary is an abnormal behavior, completely ill-adapted to human physiology, and that we must avoid as much as possible being inactive for too long. Cancer loves peace and quiet, and it is only by moving regularly that we can hope to disrupt its development.

## 3. Limit alcohol consumption

The beneficial effects of drinking small amounts of alcohol for heart health must not make us forget that this substance is very toxic in higher doses and promotes the development of several types of cancer, especially cancers of the upper digestive tract (mouth, larynx, esophagus), liver and breast. This carcinogenic effect is especially pronounced in smokers, whose risk for cancer of the buccal cavity and esophagus is increased by 40 to 60 times, which, it must be said, is another excellent reason to stop smoking.

The link between alcohol and cancer risk is still more complex in terms of breast cancer, as the consumption of any form of alcohol, even moderate (one glass a day), is associated with an increase in risk of about 10 percent. This increase in cancer risk is much lower than the reduction in risk of heart disease associated with the moderate consumption of alcoholic drinks, but drinking alcohol nonetheless remains for all women a highly personal decision that depends on each woman's comfort zone, given these risks. For those who choose to drink, it is essential to limit consumption to one glass a day to get the most benefit from alcohol's cardioprotective effect, while minimizing the risk of breast cancer or recurrence in those who have had the disease. Red wine should also be the drink of choice, owing to its positive impact on some types of cancer, especially colon cancer.

## 4. Avoid unnecessary sun exposure

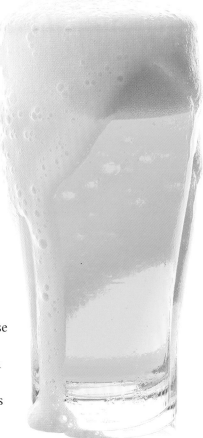

In moderation (from five to 15 minutes in the summer), exposing the skin to UV rays is very positive, as it allows the body to produce vitamin D, a substance absolutely essential for maintaining good health. When sun exposure is excessive, however, UV rays cause numerous genetic mutations to occur in skin cell DNA, which considerably increases cancer risk. The most important rule is to avoid sunburn at all costs; occasional and excessive bouts of exposure that burn the skin are the main risk factors for melanoma, especially when they occur in childhood and in fair-skinned people. In Canada, as in most industrialized countries, the incidence of skin cancer has increased dramatically in recent decades, which shows just how many people occasionally expose their skin to inordinate amounts of UV rays.

The use of sunscreens with a sun protection factor of at least 15 is therefore recommended for exposure lasting longer than 15 minutes. If you have fair skin, light-colored eyes and fair hair, use a higher SPF. But be careful: no matter what its effectiveness and protection factor, the product does not allow you to remain in the sun indefinitely. Sunscreens offering protection from both UVA and UVB rays have appeared, and these products are a very sensible option for people who have to spend long periods in the sun as part of their

activities. It is also important to note that tanning beds must be avoided totally, since studies show that very high doses of UVA rays have a cancer-causing potential as high as cigarette smoke and cause a dramatic increase in melanoma risk, especially for women.

## 5. Limit salt consumption

Public health bodies recommend a daily intake of between 1.5 and 2.4 g of sodium, which equals 3 to 6 g of salt. Most people consume much more, about 10 g of salt (4 g of sodium), and it is estimated that over two million people die prematurely from heart disease directly related to excessive sodium consumption.

Furthermore, epidemiological studies have observed that high salt consumption is correlated with a pronounced increase in the risk of stomach cancer and nasopharyngeal cancer. In Asian culinary culture, for example, salty food plays a large role (*kimchi*, *miso*, *tsukemono*s, *nuoc-mâm*), and inhabitants of Asian countries are very hard hit by these diseases, just like regions where salt has played an important historical role (Mali, Chili, Portugal).

Over 75 percent of the salt in our diet comes from industrially produced food products and is therefore consumed completely involuntarily, which exposes the population to astronomical amounts of sodium, completely out of step with what our physiology is adapted to. The only really effective way to reduce salt intake is thus to eat less of these prepared products and cook for ourselves as often as possible, so as to "wean" ourselves off the excess salt all around us. And we particularly need to remember that adding salt is not the only way to season a dish! There are several hundred different spices and herbs from the four corners of the earth, and these delicious ingredients let us explore new culinary horizons, not to mention that these plant products very often contain large amounts of molecules with many beneficial effects on health, notably for cancer prevention.

## 6. Do not take supplements to make up for a bad diet

In the West, we have developed what can only be called a supplement cult, so much so that many people would rather take vitamin C pills than eat oranges. Yet trying to condense all the healthful properties of fruits and vegetables into a single molecule is not only reductionist but also totally illogical. A simple meal, especially if you adopt the foods we have discussed, can contain several thousand vitamins, minerals and phytochemicals, as well as fiber, and it is definitely unrealistic to replace such basic food sources as plants by molecules in pills. Furthermore, several dozen studies

have clearly shown that taking supplements, whether multivitamins, selenium, large amounts of vitamin C or E, or beta-carotene, does not reduce cancer risk and is even in some cases (beta-carotene or vitamin E, for example) associated with a noticeable increase in mortality risk.

If someone's diet is deficient in vitamins, minerals and anticancer compounds because he or she does not consume enough plants, the solution to the problem does not lie in taking supplements, but rather in making major changes to eating habits. There are no miracle pills able to completely repair the damage caused by a poor-quality diet, and there never will be: you cannot eat just any old food and get away with taking a pill! With the exception of very specific medical conditions (pregnancy, severe malnutrition), supplements are not to be recommended, as they only reinforce bad eating habits and make no useful contribution to cancer prevention.

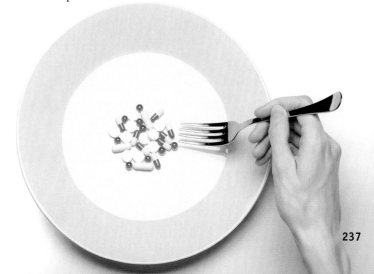

That said, there is an exception to every rule, and, in the case of supplements, the exception is vitamin D. Several studies suggest that vitamin D deficiency might encourage the development of some types of cancer, especially cancers of the colon, breast and prostate, as well as non-Hodgkin's lymphomas, and it is therefore crucial to maintain optimal levels of this vitamin. However, and contrary to other vitamins that can easily be obtained in the diet, vitamin D is quite rare in nature and is mainly produced following exposure of the skin to sunlight. This situation poses a problem for inhabitants of the planet's northern and southern regions, since the low levels of sunshine in fall and winter mean that taking supplements is really the only way to maintain adequate levels of vitamin D. For all these reasons, the Canadian Cancer Society recommends a daily intake of 1,000 IU of vitamin D in fall and winter.

## 7. Cut back on calorie intake

The only realistic approach for maintaining an ideal weight is to remove ourselves from the influence of high-calorie processed foods and adopt a diet that our metabolism has adapted to in the course of evolution — a diet mainly made up of plant products like fruits and vegetables, and whole grains. Avoid buying prepared "industrial" foods, both for snacks and main meals. These products contain far too much sugar, bad fat and salt, and are also lacking in nutritional value compared with fresh foods. Become reacquainted with your kitchen: this will ensure that you better control the amount and quality of ingredients in your diet. In addition, instead of replacing butter with margarine, use olive oil as a fat as often as possible, not just to get the benefit of its healthy fats but also because of its anticancer properties.

Finally, a simple way to reduce your calorie intake is to think of hamburgers, hot dogs, French fries, potato chips and soft drinks as occasional treats rather than daily foods. Human beings, like all animals, are very attracted by foods high in fat and sugar; eating them provides genuine pleasure that encourages repetition. It would be unrealistic to want to completely repress this instinct, but you can nonetheless turn the situation to your advantage by only eating these foods occasionally; you can then fully satisfy your cravings without the health problems associated with caloric overload.

## 8. Reduce consumption of red meat and processed meat products

Eating large amounts of red meat (beef, lamb and pork) not only increases the risk of colon cancer, but supplies enormous amounts of calories in the form of fats that can contribute to weight gain.

When meat is cooked over a flame, the fat that runs off and catches fire produces toxic compounds called aromatic hydrocarbons that stick to the meat's surface and can act as carcinogens. As well, other carcinogenic compounds called heterocyclic amines are formed by cooking animal protein at high temperature. Recent studies suggest however that marinating the meat in an acidic solution, like lemon juice, can reduce the formation of these toxic substances.

Vary your menu by using leaner meats, like chicken or fish (ideally fish high in omega-3 fats), and try to sometimes replace your daily meat with other protein sources (legumes, for example). Eating does not necessarily mean eating meat!

It is especially important to limit the consumption of processed meats and other foods containing preservation agents like nitrites — bacon, sausages, salami and ham. Several studies clearly show that these products are associated with a significant risk for colorectal cancer and shortened life expectancy. Processed meats are actually the first class of foods recognized by the World Health Organization to be Group I carcinogenic agents, meaning that their carcinogenicity has been proven in humans. Several books and Internet sites contain outstanding ideas for healthy lunches without processed meats, and these sources can be a helpful reference for people who are short of ideas. Another easy way to decrease your consumption of meat and processed meats is to rethink the role they play in daily meals. Meat does not necessarily have to be in the forefront of a dish for us to enjoy its flavor: couscous or various Asian stir-fried dishes are striking and delicious examples.

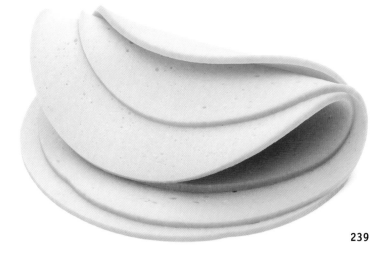

# Negative myths associated with fruits and vegetables

### Myth 1. Fruits and vegetables contain pesticides that cause cancer.

**False.** Pesticides remaining on fruits and vegetables are only found in trace amounts, and no study has been able to establish a link between these residues and cancer. On the contrary, fruit and vegetable consumption is consistently associated with a decrease in the risk of getting cancer, and there can be no doubt that the benefits of an increased intake of these foods are many times greater than the hypothetical negative effects of tiny traces of contaminants. A very simple way to eliminate almost all of these pesticide residues is to rinse your foods thoroughly with water or choose organic products.

### Myth 2. Fruits and vegetables are the product of genetic engineering, and genetically modified organisms (GMOs) are harmful to health.

**False.** The vast majority of fruits and vegetables currently available come from naturally selected varieties, without external genes introduced by humans, and can thus be considered completely natural. As for the portion of foods that really are GMOs, no study has yet established any link to cancer whatsoever, which is not very surprising since the proteins resulting from genetic modifications are in any event destroyed during digestion and cannot therefore have any real impact on nutrient intake. The problem with GMOs is above all environmental, with the most important issue being their extremely negative impact on the diversity of living plant species. This is a serious problem, and we share the concern of those who oppose them.

### Myth 3. Only "organic" fruits and vegetables are good for health.

**False.** All of the studies establishing the anticancer potential of fruits and vegetables have examined the consumption of foods grown by traditional agriculture, and it is therefore certain that the "organic" label is not an essential prerequisite for enjoying the benefits of these foods. While growing vegetables without any pesticides may stimulate the plants' defense systems, with the result that they may contain slightly higher amounts of anticancer phytochemical compounds, it is wrong to think that only these products can have positive impacts on health. It is better to eat "ordinary" fruits and vegetables daily in large amounts than to occasionally eat "organic" products whose usually higher price might cause us not to buy fruits and vegetables regularly.

## 9. Eat lots of plants

To conclude — and this is the very essence of this book — we have to increase our consumption of plants if we hope to reduce the incidence of cancer in our societies. Despite several years of programs aiming to promote increased consumption of fruits and vegetables, barely one-quarter of the current population respects the minimum recommendation of five servings a day, not to mention that the range of plants eaten is not very diverse and does not allow us to enjoy all of the benefits of these foods. This worrying situation has several causes, in particular a number of persistent myths that seem to dampen consumers' enthusiasm with respect to products of plant origin (see box, p. 240). Given the essential role of fruits and vegetables in a global cancer prevention strategy, it goes without saying that changing negative perceptions about this category of foods is an indispensable prerequisite to any significant reduction in the cancer rates currently seen in our societies.

We will say it again — there really is a close link really between a lack of plant-sourced foods, typical of the modern Western diet, and the risk of developing certain types of cancer, and we absolutely must take advantage of this relationship by changing our lifestyle habits to prevent cancer at the source before it becomes too formidable an enemy.

It is important to understand that none of the foods discussed in this book is in itself a miracle cure for cancer. This very concept of a "miracle cure," so popular in our societies, is largely responsible for people's lack of interest in the impact of their habits on the development of diseases as serious as cancer. Instead, we should approach cancer in a more realistic way and admit that in the current state of scientific and medical knowledge, this disease is too often deadly, and we must do all we can to fight its appearance by using the tools at our disposal.

We must have a fear of cancer, not a fear that paralyzes our energy or invades our thoughts, but instead a "constructive" fear that motivates us to adopt behaviors most likely to ward off the disease. Just as people can control their fear of fire by installing a smoke detector in each room in their house, we can be afraid of cancer and react by changing our behaviors so as to protect ourselves as much as possible from the disease.

As we discussed in previous chapters, this defensive approach to cancer must involve the consumption of plants that contain the largest amounts of anticancer phytochemical compounds and have been identified in population studies as having the ability to decrease the risk of several different types of cancer (Figure 92). All foods of plant origin are good for health because of their vitamin, mineral and fiber content, but only those that

| Guide to foods that fight cancer | | |
|---|---|---|
| | **Food** | **Examples** |
| Vegetables | **Cruciferous vegetables** | Broccoli, cabbage, cauliflower, Brussels sprouts, kale, radishes, turnips, cress, arugula |
| | **Garlic family** | Garlic, onions, shallots, chives, asparagus |
| | **Soy** | Miso, edamame, tofu, roasted soybeans |
| | **Tomato** | Tomato sauce, tomato paste |
| | **Mushrooms** | Shiitake, enokitake, oyster, button |
| | **Algae** | Nori, wakamé, aramé |
| Fruits | **Berries** | Blueberries, raspberries, strawberries, cranberries, blackberries, pomegranate |
| | **Citrus fruit** | Oranges, grapefruits |
| | ***Rosaceae* family** | Peaches, nectarines, plums, apples, pears, cherries |
| High-fiber foods | **Legumes** | Soybeans, black beans, lentils, peas |
| | **Grains and pasta** | Whole wheat bread and pasta, rye bread, barley, oats, buckwheat, millet |
| | **Nuts and seeds** | Sunflower seeds, almonds, pistachios |
| Good fats | **Monounsaturated** | Virgin or extra-virgin olive oil, macadamia nuts, hazelnuts, pecans, avocado |
| | **Omega-3** | Fatty fish (salmon, sardines, herring, mackerel), walnuts, flaxseeds, chia seeds |
| Seasonings | **Spices** | Turmeric, pepper, ginger, cumin, chili pepper |
| | **Herbs** | Parsley, thyme, oregano, rosemary |
| Beverages | **Green tea** | |
| | **Coffee** | |

Figure 92

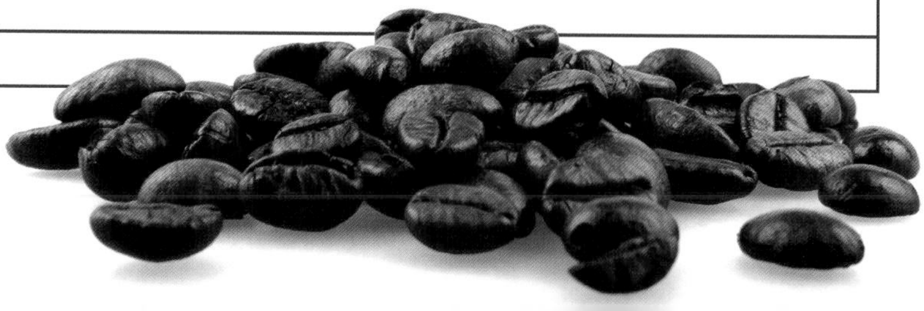

are particularly good sources of anticancer molecules can significantly reduce the risk of cancer. Regularly eating vegetables from the cabbage and garlic families, soy- and tomato-based products, fruits like berries and citrus, all enhanced with spices like turmeric and drinks like red wine, coffee and green tea can therefore be considered a form of preventive chemotherapy, in which the thousands of phytochemical compounds in these foods create an inhospitable environment for microscopic tumors and keep them in a latent and harmless state. This way of eating is based on the concepts we have tried to explain throughout this book.

## Diversity

Different classes of anticancer molecules make it possible to prevent cancer from developing by interfering in several processes involved in the disease's progression. No food contains by itself all the anticancer molecules that can act on these processes (Figure 93) — hence the importance of incorporating a wide variety of foods into eating habits. For example, eating cruciferous vegetables and vegetables from the garlic family helps the body to eliminate carcinogenic substances, thus reducing their ability to cause DNA mutations and encourage the appearance of cancer cells. Similarly,

consuming green tea, berries and soy prevents the formation of new blood vessels needed for the growth of microtumors and keeps them in a latent state. Some molecules associated with these foods even act at several stages in the cancer formation process and maximize

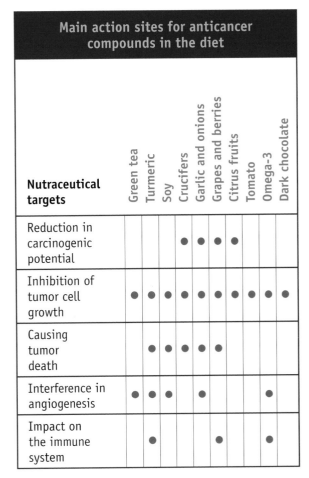

| Main action sites for anticancer compounds in the diet | | | | | | | | | |
|---|---|---|---|---|---|---|---|---|---|
| Nutraceutical targets | Green tea | Turmeric | Soy | Crucifers | Garlic and onions | Grapes and berries | Citrus fruits | Tomato | Omega-3 | Dark chocolate |
| Reduction in carcinogenic potential | | | | ● | ● | ● | ● | | | |
| Inhibition of tumor cell growth | ● | ● | ● | ● | ● | ● | ● | ● | ● | ● |
| Causing tumor death | | | ● | ● | ● | ● | ● | | | |
| Interference in angiogenesis | ● | ● | ● | | ● | | | | ● | |
| Impact on the immune system | | ● | | | | ● | | | ● | |

**Figure 93**

the protection offered by food. We just have to think of the resveratrol in grapes, which acts on all three stages in the cancerogenesis process, as well as the genistein in soy, which, in addition to being a phytoestrogen reducing the sometimes harmful effect of sex hormones, is a powerful inhibitor of several proteins involved in the uncontrolled growth of cancer cells. The diversity of anticancer molecules in the diet is important, as cancer cells use many tricks to grow, and it is definitely unrealistic to think their ability to overcome obstacles can be controlled by using anticancer molecules that interfere with just one process. We must emphasize again the central role of soy, green tea and turmeric; these foods are beyond a doubt major preventive tools that contribute to the huge differences between cancer rates in the East and West.

To make a simple analogy, if you carry a pail of water with holes in it to several places, plugging a few holes will not keep the water from leaking out — you have to plug all the holes. The same is true of cancer: only by attacking it on several fronts can we hope to succeed in preventing it from escaping and reaching its full maturity.

## Moderation and regularity

Regular absorption of these anticancer phytochemical molecules is necessary to keep precancerous cells off balance and prevent them from growing. This idea of continual combat is very important: since we all have immature tumors, we must think of cancer as a chronic disease requiring constant treatment to keep it in a latent state. This is true both for people who want to avoid getting cancer and for survivors of the disease: the anticancer molecules in these foods slow down the progression of microscopic tumors that form spontaneously during our lives, and several studies suggest that they could even do the same for microtumor sites that have not been completely eliminated by surgical, radiotherapy or chemotherapy treatments.

The first reflex of some people who become aware of the essential role of diet in cancer prevention will often be to think that the greater the amount of anticancer foods consumed, the greater the benefits. They may decide to combine all of the foods described in this book, in a blender for example, to create

## Nutraprevention: Fruits and vegetables

- Increase consumption
- Vary consumption
- Choose dishes made up of several varieties
- Eat them daily

anticancer "cocktails" containing extraordinary amounts of fruits and vegetables impossible to reach if these foods were eaten in their natural solid form. This extremely aggressive approach is not realistic, however; this kind of medicalization of the diet destroys our special relationship with food and cannot be sustained in the long term because of its monotony and the lack of enjoyment associated with it. In other words, there is no point in eating an extravagant meal once a week containing enormous amounts of the foods described in this book, while ignoring these foods the rest of the time. This way of thinking contributes nothing really useful to any cancer prevention effort, any more than the injection of a massive dose of insulin solves a diabetic's blood sugar problems in the long run.

It is often said that moderation is the basis of a healthy diet, and the same is true for all efforts related to cancer prevention: preventing cancer through diet must be seen as a constant and steady task that can only be accomplished by changing eating habits to incorporate as often as possible a wide variety of plants with the strongest anticancer activities. These changes are not at all radical or extreme; in every study, it is moderate consumption of anticancer foods two to four times a week that has been associated with a decrease in cancer risk. It is just a matter of regaining control over our daily diet, reconsidering its place in

our lives and looking at it not as an act solely designed to satisfy our essential needs, but also as a major contribution to our overall well-being.

The Mediterranean diet illustrates this concept very well, as shown by the results obtained in the Spanish clinical study PREDIMED (PREvención con DIeta MEDiterránea), started in 2003 to determine the influence of this diet on heart disease. The participants in this random clinical study were divided into three groups: 1) a Mediterranean diet supplemented with extra-virgin olive oil; 2) a Mediterranean diet supplemented with a mixture of nuts; and 3) a low-fat diet, as suggested by heart disease organizations. When the incidence of breast cancer in 4,152 women aged 60 to 80 who participated in the study was examined, it was noticed that those who followed a Mediterranean diet were much less affected by cancer, with a decrease in risk of 40 percent in the group whose diet was supplemented by a mixture of nuts and 70 percent in the group whose diet was supplemented by extra-virgin olive oil (Figure 94). Since random trials are considered to be the gold standard in clinical research (the subjects are divided randomly, to minimize statistical distortion), the dramatic decrease in breast cancer risk observed is one of the best proofs to date of the key role played by diet in cancer prevention.

## Effectiveness

As we have seen, anticancer agents in food are often able to act directly on a tumor and limit its development, both by causing the death of cancer cells and by preventing it from progressing to more advanced stages — by interfering with the formation of a new blood vessel network or by stimulating the organism's immune defenses, for example (Figure 95).

The combination of several foods, however, all containing different anticancer compounds, makes it possible not only to target different processes associated with tumor growth, but also to make their action more effective. In fact, thanks to this synergy, a molecule's anticancer action can be considerably increased by the presence of another molecule, a very important property for compounds in food, which are usually present in small amounts in the blood. For example, neither curcumin nor the main polyphenol in green tea, EGCG, is able on its own to cause cancer cell death when present in small amounts. On the other hand, when these two molecules are added at the same time, they cause a very significant response that results in the death of cells by apoptosis (Figure 96). This kind of direct synergy can also considerably increase the therapeutic response to a specific anticancer treatment. For example, research in our laboratory has shown that adding curcumin and EGCG to cancer cells subjected to low doses of radiation causes a spectacular increase in the response of these cells to treatment (same figure).

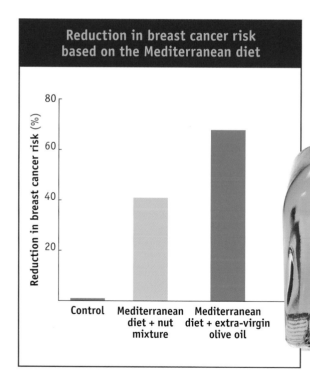

**Reduction in breast cancer risk based on the Mediterranean diet**

Reduction in breast cancer risk (%)

**Figure 94**

Adapted from Toledo et al., 2015.

Synergy also often relies on indirect mechanisms. For example, the foods we eat daily contain a wide range of molecules with no anticancer activity of their own, but these molecules may have a considerable impact on cancer prevention by increasing the amount (and thus the anticancer potential) of another anticancer molecule in the blood, either by slowing down its elimination or by enhancing its absorption (Figure 95). One of the best examples of this indirect synergy is the property of a molecule in pepper, piperine, to increase by more than 1,000 the absorption of curcumin (Figure 97), making it possible to attain levels of curcumin in the blood likely to really change the aggressive behavior of cancer cells. In our opinion, not only does this synergy illustrate the need to adopt a varied diet to maximize its health benefits, but it also makes replacing foods with pure molecules in supplement form totally illogical.

## Eating for health and enjoying it

The search for health benefits must not be at the expense of gastronomic enjoyment; on the contrary, it must be part of the same preventive perspective. This is an important notion, for we must get real pleasure out of healthy eating to

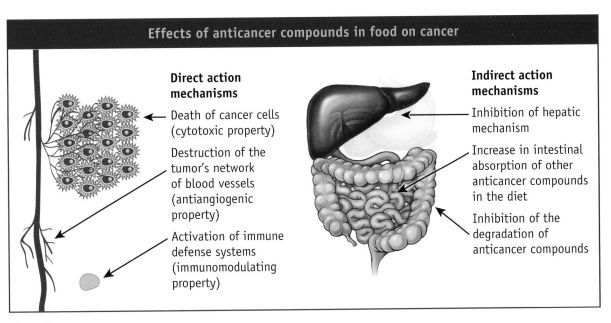

**Effects of anticancer compounds in food on cancer**

**Direct action mechanisms**

Death of cancer cells (cytotoxic property)

Destruction of the tumor's network of blood vessels (antiangiogenic property)

Activation of immune defense systems (immunomodulating property)

**Indirect action mechanisms**

Inhibition of hepatic mechanism

Increase in intestinal absorption of other anticancer compounds in the diet

Inhibition of the degradation of anticancer compounds

**Figure 95**

feed ourselves well every day. Preventing cancer through diet can become a very pleasant activity when we treat it as if we were preparing a feast! The simplest way, and what we advise you to do, is to collect a few books of basic recipes from different culinary traditions that use the foods mentioned in this book. There is no point in reinventing the wheel: the peoples of the Middle East have been cooking legumes for at least 3,000 years and have acquired considerable know-how in preparing these dishes. Asian cooking offers many possible ways to use soy in every form, and you will find the best ways to cook this food in these books, not to mention the systematic use by these various traditions of many healthy vegetables, especially the different varieties of cabbage. The Mediterranean peoples and the Japanese have elevated the preparation of fish and seafood to an art and are an essential reference to guide you in preparing this kind of meal. The same is true for the Italians and Spanish in the case of tomatoes, or Indian cooking for various curries.

These recipes offer a golden opportunity to cook delicious meals while drawing on the principles we have discussed in this book. This is

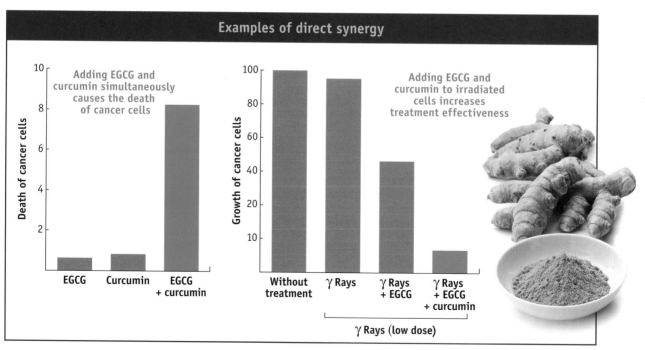

**Figure 96**

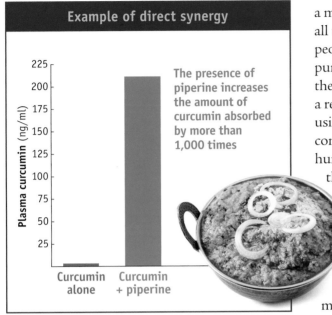

**Example of direct synergy**

The presence of piperine increases the amount of curcumin absorbed by more than 1,000 times

Plasma curcumin (ng/ml)

Curcumin alone / Curcumin + piperine

**Figure 97**

a major point, for healthy eating means above all taking real pleasure in eating. For most people, a diet is something boring, a synonym for punishment and deprivation. On the contrary, the program we are suggesting must be viewed as a reward! Having access to thousands of recipes using healthy and delicious ingredients, and constantly varying your meals to include the hundreds of fruits and vegetables available on the market, is much more like epicureanism than self-denial. The astonishing wealth of practical knowledge passed on from generation to generation is the most wonderful experiment ever carried out on earth, a priceless legacy that embodies our species' endless quest to make the most of the riches nature offers for our own health and enjoyment.

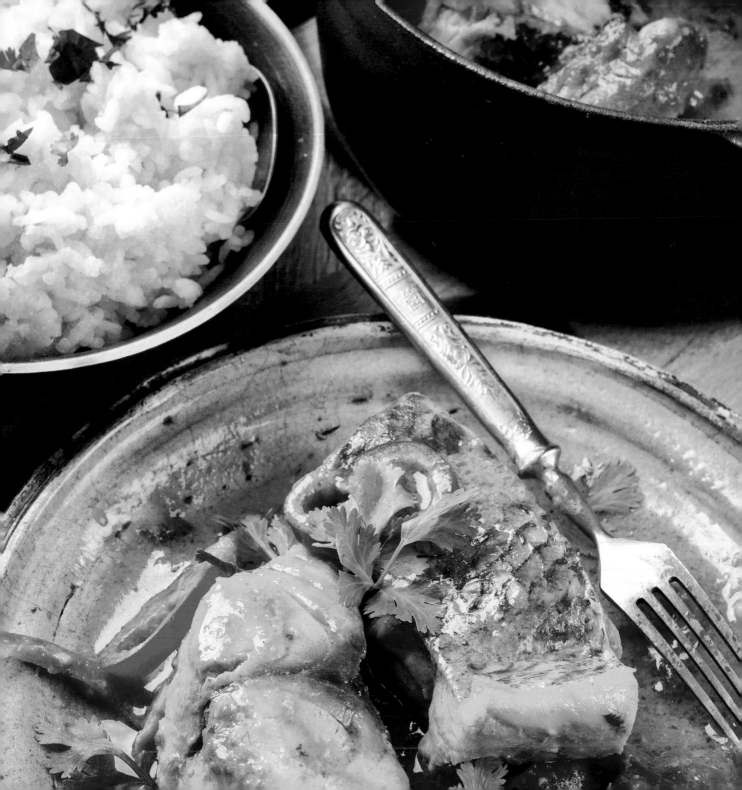

# Conclusion

Changing our diet to incorporate certain foods that are exceptional sources of anticancer molecules is one of the best weapons currently at our disposal for fighting cancer.

These changes in habit are not at all extreme or revolutionary: it is simply a matter of restoring food to its important role in daily life by paying more attention to the consequences that the food we eat can have on our overall well-being. You can take enormous satisfaction from putting these changes into practice, both for the gastronomic enjoyment they offer and for the feeling of satisfaction you get from participating actively in your body's defense mechanisms by providing it daily with a large dose of nutraceuticals. Using the plentiful food resources we have the immense privilege to have access to, not only to feed ourselves but also to reduce the incidence of diseases as serious as cancer, could be one of the most important advances in our fight against this disease.

Cuisine is the culture of humanity, the expression of our ingenuity in exploring our environment and discovering new foods, the illustration of our constant quest for well-being. It is impossible to resign ourselves to the idea that barely one century of industrialization should succeed in destroying this heritage and, in so doing, deny the collective knowledge of humanity and lay waste its fundamental principles. Preventing cancer through diet is thus above all about recapturing the essence of the food culture developed over millennia by civilizations. It is about paying homage to the priceless knowledge acquired by thousands of generations of people who wanted to give their children the foods needed for good health, while seeking the best way to prepare these foods so they would be enjoyed. It is about paying respect to humanity's most amazing accomplishment, without which we would not exist. Preventing cancer through diet is simply about reconnecting with the very essence of the human condition.

## Chapter 1

Siegel, R. et coll. "Cancer statistics, 2014", *CA Cancer J Clin* 2014; 64: 9-29.

Lichtenstein, P. et coll. "Environmental and heritable factors in the causation of cancer – analyses of cohorts of twins from Sweden, Denmark, and Finland", *N Engl J Med* 2000; 343: 78-85.

Greaves, M.F. "Leukemia in twins: lessons in natural history", *Blood* 2003; 102: 2321-33.

Sørensen, T.I. et coll. "Genetic and environmental influences on premature death in adult adoptees", *N Engl J Med* 1988; 318: 727-732.

King, M.C. et coll. "Breast and ovarian cancer risks due to inherited mutations in BRCA1 and BRCA2", *Science* 2003; 302: 643-6.

Nkondjock, A. et coll. "Diet, lifestyle and BRCA-related breast cancer risk among French-Canadians", *Breast Cancer Res Treat* 2006; 98: 285-294.

Doll, R. et R. Peto. "The causes of cancer: Quantitative estimates of avoidable risks of cancer in the United States today", *J Natl Cancer Inst* 1981; 66: 1196-1265.

Kuriki, K. et K. Tajima. "The increasing incidence of colorectal cancer and the preventive strategy in Japan", *Asian Pacific J Cancer Prev* 2006; 7: 495-501.

*AACR Cancer Progress Report 2011*, https://www.roswellpark.org/sites/default/files/node-files/asset/nid91575-2011-aacr-cpr-text-web.pdf.

World Cancer Research Fund/American Institute of Cancer Research, "Food, Nutrition, Physical Activity and the Prevention of Cancer: a Global Perspective", http://www.dietandcancerreport.org.

Platz, E.A. et coll. "Proportion of colon cancer risk that might be preventable in a cohort of middle-aged US men", *Cancer Causes Control* 2000; 11: 579-88.

Cordain, L. et coll. "Origins and evolution of the Western diet: health implications for the 21st century", *Am J Clin Nutr* 2005; 81: 341-354.

Weil, A. *Le guide essentiel de la diététique et de la santé*, Paris, J'ai lu, 2000, 414 pages.

Willett, W.C. *Eat, Drink and Be Healthy: The Harvard Medical School Guide to Healthy Eating*, New York, Free Press, 2001.

## Chapter 2

Weinberg, R.A. *One Renegade Cell: How Cancer Begins*, New York, Basic Books, 1998.

Weinstein, I.B. "The origins of human cancer: molecular mechanisms of carcinogenesis and their implications for cancer prevention and treatment – Twenty-seventh G.H.A. Clowes Memorial Award Lecture", *Cancer Res* 1988; 48: 4135-43.

Sonnenschein, C. et A.M. Soto. "The death of the cancer cell", *Cancer Res* 2011; 71: 4334-7.

Cho, K.R. et B. Vogelstein. "Genetic alterations in the adenoma-carcinoma sequence", *Cancer* 1992; 70 (Suppl): 1727-31.

Hanahan, D. et R.A. Weinberg. "The hallmarks of cancer", *Cell* 2000; 100: 57-70.

Greaves, M. "Darwinian medicine: a case for cancer", *Nature Rev Cancer* 2007; 7: 213-221.

Vogelstein, B. et coll. "Cancer genome landscapes", *Science* 2013; 339: 1546-58.

Gottesman, M.M. "Mechanisms of cancer drug resistance", *Annu Rev Med* 2002; 53: 615-27.

Curtis, C. et coll. "The genomic and transcriptomic architecture of 2,000 breast tumours reveals novel subgroups", *Nature* 2012; 486: 346-52.

de Bruin, E.C. et coll. "Spatial and temporal diversity in genomic instability processes defines lung cancer evolution", *Science* 2014; 346: 251-6.

## Chapter 3

Bissell, M.J. et W.C. Hines. "Why don't we get more cancer? A proposed role of the microenvironment in restraining cancer progression", *Nat Med* 2011; 17: 320-9.

Folkman, J. "Angiogenesis in cancer, vascular, rheumatoid and other diseases", *Nature Med* 1995; 1: 27-31.

Tosetti, F. et coll. "Angioprevention: angiogenesis is a common and key target for cancer chemopreventive agents", *FASEB J.* 2002; 16: 2-14.

Coussens, L.M. et Z. Werb. "Inflammation and cancer", *Nature* 2002; 420: 860-867.

Balkwill, F. et L.M. Coussens. "Cancer: an inflammatory link", *Nature* 2004; 431: 405-6.

Karin, M. "Nuclear factor-kappaB in cancer development and progression", *Nature* 2006; 441: 431-6.

De Visser, K.E. et L.M. Coussens. "The inflammatory tumor microenvironment and its impact on cancer development", *Contrib Microbiol* 2006; 13: 118-37.

Balkwill, F. et coll. "Smoldering and polarized inflammation in the initiation and promotion of malignant disease", *Cancer Cell* 2005; 7: 211-7.

Finak, G. et coll. "Stromal gene expression predicts clinical outcome in breast cancer", *Nat Med* 2008; 14: 518-27.

Kopelman, P.G. "Obesity as a medical problem", *Nature* 2000; 404: 635-43.

Hummasti, S. et G.S. Hotamisligil. "Endoplasmic reticulum stress and inflammation in obesity and diabetes", *Circ Res* 2010; 107: 579-91.

Calle, E.E. et R. Kaaks. "Overweight, obesity and cancer: epidemiological evidence and proposed mechanisms", *Nature Rev Cancer* 2004; 4: 579-591.

Khandekar, M.J. et coll. "Molecular mechanisms of cancer development in obesity", *Nat Rev Cancer* 2011; 11: 886-95.

Williams, S.C.P. "Link between obesity and cancer", *Proc Natl Acad Sci USA* 2013; 110: 8753-54.

Arnold, M. et coll. "Global burden of cancer attributable to high body-mass index in 2012: a population-based study", *Lancet Oncol* 2015; 16: 36-46.

Brown, L.M. et coll. "Incidence of adenocarcinoma of the esophagus among white Americans by sex, stage, and age", *J Natl Cancer Inst* 2008; 100: 1184-7.

## Chapter 4

Ungar, P.S. et M.F. Teaford, dirs. *Human Diet: Its Origin and Evolution*, Westport (CT), Praeger, 2002, 192 pages.

Stahl, A.B. et coll. "Hominid dietary selection before fire [and comments and reply]", *Current Anthropology* 1984; 25: 151-168.

Proches, S. et coll. "Plant diversity in the human diet: Weak phylogenetic signal indicates breadth", *Bioscience* 2008; 58: 151-159.

Hardy, K. et coll. "Neanderthal medics? Evidence for food, cooking, and medicinal plants entrapped in dental calculus", *Naturwissenschaften* 2012; 99: 617-26.

Cragg, G.M. et D.J. Newman. "Plants as a source of anti-cancer agents", *J Ethnopharmacol* 2005; 100: 72-9.

Corson, T.W. et C.M. Crews. "Molecular understanding and modern application of traditional medicines: triumphs and trials", *Cell* 2007; 130: 769-74.

Black, W.C. et H.G. Welch. "Advances in diagnostic imaging and overestimation of disease prevalence and the benefits of therapy", *N Engl J Med* 1993; 328: 1237-1243.

Folkman, J. et R. Kalluri. "Cancer without disease", *Nature* 2004; 427: 787.

Nielsen, M. et coll. "Breast cancer and atypia among young and middle-aged women: a study of 110 medicolegal autopsies", *Br J Cancer* 1987; 56: 814-9

Sakr, W.A. et coll. "The frequency of carcinoma and intraepithelial neoplasia of the prostate in young male patients", *J Urol* 1993; 150: 379-385.

Watanabe, M. et coll. "Comparative studies of prostate cancer in Japan versus the United States. A review", *Urol Oncol* 2000; 5: 274-283.

London, S.J. et coll. "Isothiocyanates, glutathione S-transferase M1 and T1 polymorphisms, and lung-cancer risk: a prospective study of men in Shanghai, China", *Lancet* 2000; 356: 724-729.

Boivin, D. et coll. "Antiproliferative and antioxidant activities of common vegetables: A comparative study", *Food Chem* 2009; 112: 374-380.

Boivin, D. et coll. "Inhibition of cancer cell proliferation and suppression of TNF-induced activation of NFkappaB by edible berry juice", *Anticancer Res* 2007; 27: 937-48.

McCullough, M.L. et E.L. Giovannucci. "Diet and cancer prevention", *Oncogene* 2004; 23: 6349-6364.

Key, T.J. et coll. "The effect of diet on risk of cancer", *Lancet* 2002; 360: 861-868.

## Chapter 5

Manach, C. et coll. "Polyphenols: food sources and bioavailability", *Am J Clin Nutr* 2004; 79: 727-747.

Bode, A.M. et Z. Dong. "Targeting signal transduction pathways by chemopreventive agents", *Mut Res* 2004; 555: 33-51.

Anand, P. et coll. "Cancer is a preventable disease that requires major lifestyle changes", *Pharm Res* 2008; 25: 2097-116.

The ATBC Study Group. "The effect of vitamin E and beta-carotene on the incidence of lung cancer and other cancers in male smokers", *N Engl J Med* 1994; 330: 1029-1035.

Miller, E.R. et coll. "High-dosage vitamin E supplementation may increase all-cause mortality", *Ann Intern Med* 2005; 142: 37-46.

Klein, E.A. et coll. "Vitamin E and the risk of prostate cancer: the Selenium and Vitamin E Cancer Prevention Trial (SELECT)", *JAMA* 2011; 306: 1549-56.

Kristal, A.R. et coll. "Baseline selenium status and effects of selenium and vitamin E supplementation on prostate cancer risk", *J Natl Cancer Inst* 2014; 106: djt456.

Mithöfer, A. et W. Boland. "Plant defense against herbivores: chemical aspects", *Annu Rev Plant Biol* 2012; 63: 431-50.

Hare, J.D. "Ecological role of volatiles produced by plants in response to damage by herbivorous insects", *Annu Rev Entomol* 2011; 56: 161-80.

Hughes, S. "Antelope activate the acacia's alarm system", *New Scientist* 1990; 1736: 19.

Béliveau, R. et D. Gingras. "Role of nutrition in preventing cancer", *Can Fam Physician* 2007; 53: 1905-11.

Cho, I. et M.J. Blaser. "The human microbiome: at the interface of health and disease", *Nat Rev Genet* 2012; 13: 260-70.

Smith, P.M. et coll. "The microbial metabolites, short-chain fatty acids, regulate colonic Treg cell homeostasis", *Science* 2013; 341: 569-573.

Roopchand, D.E. et coll. "Dietary polyphenols promote growth of the gut bacterium and attenuate high fat diet-induced metabolic syndrome", *Diabetes* 2015 Apr 6. pii: db141916.

Drewnowski, A. et C. Gomez-Carneros. "Bitter taste, phytonutrients, and the consumer: a review", *Am J Clin Nutr* 2000; 72: 1424-35.

Hung, H.C. et coll. "Fruit and vegetable intake and risk of major chronic disease", *J Natl Cancer Inst* 2004; 96: 1577-84.

Boffetta, P. et coll. "Fruit and vegetable intake and overall cancer risk in the European Prospective Investigation into Cancer and Nutrition (EPIC)", *J Natl Cancer Inst* 2010; 102: 529-37.

Fung, T.T. et coll. "Intake of specific fruits and vegetables in relation to risk of estrogen receptor-negative breast cancer among postmenopausal women", *Breast Cancer Res Treat* 2013; 138: 925-30.

Stevenson, D.E. et R.D. Hurst. "Polyphenolic phytochemicals – just antioxidants or much more?", *Cell Mol Life Sci* 2007; 64: 2900-16.

Eberhardt, M.V. et coll. "Antioxidant activity of fresh apples", *Nature* 2000; 405: 903-4.

Surh, Y.J. "Cancer chemoprevention with dietary phytochemicals", *Nature Rev Cancer* 2003; 3: 768-780.

Dorai, T. et B.B. Aggarwal. "Role of chemopreventive agents in cancer therapy", *Cancer Lett* 2004; 215: 129-140.

## Chapter 6

Hedge, I.C. "A systematic and geographical survey of the Old World Cruciferae", dans Vaughn, J.G., A.J. Macleod et B.M.G. Jones, dirs. *The Biology and Chemistry of the Cruciferae*, Londres, Academic Press, 1976, p. 1-45.

Wright, C.A. *Mediterranean Vegetables: A Cook's ABC of Vegetables and Their Preparation in Spain, France, Italy, Greece, Turkey, the Middle East, and North Africa with More Than 200 Authentic Recipes for the Home Cook*, Boston (MA), Harvard Common Press, 2001, p. 77-79.

Michaud, D.S. et coll. "Fruit and vegetable intake and incidence of bladder cancer in a male prospective cohort", *J Natl Cancer Inst* 1999; 91: 605-13.

Terry, P. et coll. "Brassica vegetables and breast cancer risk", *JAMA* 2001; 285: 2975-2977.

Wu, Q.J. et coll. "Cruciferous vegetables consumption and the risk of female lung cancer: a prospective study and a meta-analysis", *Ann Oncol* 2013; 24: 1918-1924.

Kirsh, V.A. et coll. "Prospective study of fruit and vegetable intake and risk of prostate cancer", *J Natl Cancer Inst* 2007; 99: 1200-9.

Moy, K.A. "Isothiocyanates, glutathione S-transferase M1 and T1 polymorphisms and gastric cancer risk: a prospective study of men in Shanghai, China", *Int J Cancer* 2009; 125: 2652-9.

Suzuki, R. et coll. "Fruit and vegetable intake and breast cancer risk defined by estrogen and progesterone receptor status: the Japan Public Health Center-based Prospective Study", *Cancer Causes Control* 2013; 24: 2117-28.

Wu, Q.J. et coll. "Cruciferous vegetables intake and the risk of colorectal cancer: a meta-analysis of observational studies", *Ann Oncol* 2013; 24: 1079-87.

Tang, L. et coll. "Intake of cruciferous vegetables modifies bladder cancer survival", *Cancer Epidemiol Biomarkers Prev* 2010; 19: 1806-11.

Thomson, C.A. et coll. "Vegetable intake is associated with reduced breast cancer recurrence in tamoxifen users: a secondary analysis from the Women's Healthy Eating and Living Study", *Breast Cancer Res Treat* 2011; 125: 519-527.

Verhoeven, D.T.H. et coll. "Epidemiological studies on Brassica vegetables and cancer risk", *Cancer Epidemiol Biomarkers Prev* 1996; 5: 733-748.

Talalay, P. et J.W. Fahey. "Phytochemicals from cruciferous plants protect against cancer by modulating carcinogen metabolism", *J Nutr* 2001; 131: 3027S-3033S.

Keum, Y.S. et coll. "Chemoprevention by isothiocyanates and their underlying molecular signaling mechanisms", *Mut Res* 2004; 555: 191-202.

Johnston, C.S. et coll. "More Americans are eating "5 a day" but intakes of dark green and cruciferous vegetables remain low", *J Nutr* 2000; 130: 3063-3067.

Fenwick, G.R. et coll. "Glucosinolates and their breakdown products in food and food plants", *CRC Critical Rev Food Sci and Nutr* 1983; 18: 123-201.

Jones, R.B. et coll. "Cooking method significantly effects glucosinolate content and sulforaphane production in broccoli florets", *Food Chem* 2010; 123: 237-242.

Mullaney, J.A. et coll. "Lactic acid bacteria convert glucosinolates to nitriles efficiently yet differently from enterobacteriaceae", *J Agric Food Chem* 2013; 61: 3039-46.

McNaughton, S.A. et G.C. Marks. "Development of a food composition database for the estimation of dietary intakes of glucosinolates, the biologically active constituents of cruciferous vegetables", *Br J Nutr* 2003; 90: 687-697.

Zhang, Y. et coll. "A major inducer of anticarcinogenic protective enzymes from broccoli: isolation and elucidation of structure", *Proc Natl Acad Sci USA* 1992; 89: 2399-2403.

Fahey, J.W. et coll. "Broccoli sprouts: an exceptionally rich source of inducers of enzymes that protect against chemical carcinogens", *Proc Natl Acad Sci USA* 1997; 94: 10367-10372.

Lenzi, M. et coll. "Sulforaphane as a promising molecule for fighting cancer", *Cancer Treat Res* 2014; 159: 207-23.

Gingras, D. et coll. "Induction of medulloblastoma cell apoptosis by sulforaphane, a dietary anticarcinogen from Brassica vegetables", *Cancer Lett* 2004; 203: 35-43.

Fahey, J.W. et coll. "Sulforaphane inhibits extracellular, intracellular and antibiotic-resistant strains of *Helicobacter pylori* and prevents benzo[a]pyrene-induces stomach tumors", *Proc Natl Acad Sci USA* 2002; 99: 7610-7615.

Hecht, S.S. et coll. "Effects of watercress consumption on metabolism of a tobacco-specific lung carcinogen in smokers", *Cancer Epidemiol Biomarkers Prev* 1995; 4: 877-84.

Qin, C.Z. et coll. "Advances in molecular signaling mechanisms of β-phenethyl isothiocyanate antitumor effects", *J Agric Food Chem* 2015; 63: 3311-22.

Wang, D. et coll. "Phenethyl isothiocyanate upregulates death receptors 4 and 5 and inhibits proliferation in human cancer stem-like cells", *BMC Cancer* 2014; 14: 591.

Bradlow, H.L. et coll. "Multifunctional aspects of the action of indole-3-carbinol as an antitumor agent", *Ann NY Acad Sci* 1999; 889: 204-213.

## Chapter 7

Block, E. "The chemistry of garlic and onion", *Sci Am* 1985; 252: 114-119.

Rivlin, R.S. "Historical perspective on the use of garlic", *J Nutr* 2001; 131: 951S-4S.

Lawson, L.D. et Z.J. Wang. "Low allicin release from garlic supplements: a major problem due to the sensitivities of alliinase activity", *J Agric Food Chem* 2001; 49: 2592-9.

Imai, S. et coll. "An onion enzyme that makes the eyes water", *Nature* 2002; 419: 685.

Milner, J.A. "A historical perspective on garlic and cancer", *J Nutr* 2001; 131: 1027S-31S.

Nicastro, H.L. et coll. "Garlic and onions: their cancer prevention properties", *Cancer Prev Res* 2015; 8: 181-9.

Zhou, Y. et coll. "Consumption of large amounts of Allium vegetables reduces risk for gastric cancer in a metaanalysis", *Gastroenterology* 2011; 141: 80-9.

Gonzalez, C.A. et coll. "Fruit and vegetable intake and the risk of stomach and œsophagus adenocarcinoma in the European Prospective Investigation into Cancer and Nutrition (EPIC-EURGAST)", *Int J Cancer* 2006; 118: 2559-2566.

Galeone, C. et coll. "Onion and garlic use and human cancer", *Am J Clin Nutr* 2006; 84: 1027-32.

Zhou, X.F. et coll. "Allium vegetables and risk of prostate cancer: evidence from 132,192 subjects", *Asian Pac J Cancer Prev* 2013; 14: 4131-4.

Millen, A.E. et coll. "Fruit and vegetable intake and prevalence of colorectal adenoma in a cancer screening trial", *Am J Clin Nutr* 2007; 86: 1754-64.

Gao, C.M. et coll. "Protective effect of allium vegetables against both œsophageal and stomach cancer: a simultaneous case-referent study of a high-epidemic area in Jiangsu Province, China", *Jpn J Cancer Res* 1999; 90: 614-21.

Buiatti, E. et coll. "A case-control study of gastric cancer and diet in Italy", *Int J Cancer* 1989; 44: 611-6.

Hsing, A.W. et coll. "Allium vegetables and risk of prostate cancer: a population-based study", *J Natl Cancer Inst* 2002; 94: 1648-51.

Gonzalez, C.A. et coll. "Fruit and vegetable intake and the risk of stomach and œsophagus adenocarcinoma in the European Prospective Investigation into Cancer and Nutrition (EPIC-EURGAST)", *Int J Cancer* 2006; 118: 2559-2566.

Gao, C.M. et coll. "Protective effect of allium vegetables against both œsophageal and stomach cancer: a simultaneous case-referent study of a high-epidemic area in Jiangsu Province, China", *Jap J Cancer Res* 1999; 90: 614-621.

Steinmetz, K.A. et coll. "Vegetables, fruit, and colon cancer in the Iowa Women's Health Study", *Am J Epidemiol* 1994; 139: 1-15.

Challier, B. et coll. "Garlic, onion and cereal fibre as protective factors for breast cancer: a French case-control study", *Eur J Epidemiol* 1998; 14: 737-747.

Yi, L. et Q. Su. "Molecular mechanisms for the anti-cancer effects of diallyl disulfide", *Food Chem Toxicol* 2013; 57: 362-70.

Herman-Antosiewicz, A. et S.V. Singh. "Signal transduction pathways leading to cell cycle arrest and apoptosis induction in cancer cells by Allium vegetable-derived organosulfur compounds: a review", *Mut Res* 2004; 555: 121-131.

Milner, J.A. "Mechanisms by which garlic and allyl sulfur compounds suppress carcinogen bioactivation. Garlic and carcinogenesis", *Adv Exp Med Biol* 2001; 492: 69-81.

Yang, C.S. et coll. "Mechanisms of inhibition of chemical toxicity and carcinogenesis by diallyl sulfide (DAS) and related compounds from garlic", *J Nutr* 2001; 131: 1041S-5S.

Demeule, M. et coll. "Diallyl disulfide, a chemopreventive agent in garlic, induces multidrug resistance-associated protein 2 expression", *Biochem Biophys Res Commun* 2004; 324: 937-45.

## Chapter 8

Shurtleff, W. et A. Aoyagi. *History of Whole Dry Soybeans, Used as Beans, or Ground, Mashed or Flaked (240 BCE to 2013)*, California, Lafayette, 1980, 950 pages.

Clemons, M. et P. Goss. "Estrogen and the risk of breast cancer", *N Engl J Med* 2001; 344: 276-285.

Setchell, K.D. "Phytoestrogens: the biochemistry, physiology, and implications for human health of soy isoflavones", *Am J Clin Nutr* 1998; 68: 1333S-1346S.

Magee, P.J. et I.R. Rowland. "Phyto-œstrogens, their mechanism of action: current evidence for a role in breast and prostate cancer", *Br J Nutr* 2004; 91: 513-531.

Sarkar, F.H. et Y. Li. "Mechanisms of cancer chemoprevention by soy isoflavone genistein", *Cancer Metast Rev* 2002; 21: 265-280.

Lee, H.P. et coll. "Dietary effects on breast cancer risk in Singapore", *Lancet* 1991; 331: 1197-1200.

Yamamoto, S. et coll. "Soy, isoflavones, and breast cancer risk in Japan", *J Natl Cancer Inst* 2003; 95: 906-913.

Horn-Ross, P.L. et coll. "Recent diet and breast cancer risk: the California Teachers Study (USA)", *Cancer Causes Control* 2002; 13: 407-15.

Messina, M. et coll. "Estimated Asian adult soy protein and isoflavone intakes", *Nutr Cancer* 2006; 55: 1-12.

Lee, S.A. et coll. "Adolescent and adult soy food intake and breast cancer risk: results from the Shanghai Women's Health Study", *Am J Clin Nutr* 2009; 89: 1920-6.

Warri, A. et coll. "The role of early life genistein exposures in modifying breast cancer risk", *Br J Cancer* 2008; 98: 1485-93.

Lamartiniere, C.A. et coll. "Genistein chemoprevention: timing and mechanisms of action in murine mammary and prostate", *J Nutr* 2002; 132: 552S-558S.

Severson, R.K. et coll. "A prospective study of demographics, diet, and prostate cancer among men of Japanese ancestry in Hawaii", *Cancer Res* 1989; 49: 1857-60.

Jacobsen, B.K. et coll. "Does high soy milk intake reduce prostate cancer incidence? The Adventist Health Study", *Cancer Causes Control* 1998; 9: 553-7.

Kurahashi, N. et coll. "Plasma isoflavones and subsequent risk of prostate cancer in a nested case-control study: the Japan Public Health Center", *J Clin Oncol* 2008; 26: 5923-9.

Chen, M. et coll. "Association between soy isoflavone intake and breast cancer risk for pre- and post-menopausal women: a meta-analysis of epidemiological studies", *PLoS One* 2014; 9: e89288.

Ollberding, N.J. et coll. "Legume, soy, tofu, and isoflavone intake and endometrial cancer risk in postmenopausal women in the multiethnic cohort study", *J Natl Cancer Inst* 2012; 104: 67-76.

Yang, W.S. et coll. "Soy intake is associated with lower lung cancer risk: results from a meta-analysis of epidemiologic studies", *Am J Clin Nutr* 2011; 94: 1575-83.

Schabath, M.B. et coll. "Dietary phytoestrogens and lung cancer risk", *JAMA* 2005; 294: 1493-504.

Allred, C.D. et coll. "Soy processing influences growth of estrogen-dependent breast cancer tumor", *Carcinogenesis* 2004; 25: 1649-1657.

Fritz, H. et coll. "Soy, red clover, and isoflavones and breast cancer: a systematic review", *PLoS One* 2013; 8: e81968.

Adlercreutz, H. et coll. "Dietary phytoœstrogens and the menopause in Japan", *Lancet* 1992; 339: 1233.

Rossouw, J.E. et coll. "Risks and benefits of estrogen plus progestin in healthy postmenopausal women: principal results from the Women's Health Initiative randomized controlled trial", *JAMA* 2002; 288: 321-33.

Guha, N. et coll. "Soy isoflavones and risk of cancer recurrence in a cohort of breast cancer survivors: the Life After Cancer Epidemiology study", *Breast Cancer Res Treat* 2009; 118: 395-405.

Shu, X.O. et coll. "Soy food intake and breast cancer survival", *JAMA* 2009; 302: 2437-2443.

Chi, F. et coll. "Post-diagnosis soy food intake and breast cancer survival: a meta-analysis of cohort studies", *Asian Pac J Cancer Prev* 2013; 14: 2407-12.

Nechuta, S.J. et coll. "Soy food intake after diagnosis of breast cancer and survival: an in-depth analysis of combined evidence from cohort studies of US and Chinese women", *Am J Clin Nutr* 2012; 96: 123-32.

Kang, X. et coll. "Effect of soy isoflavones on breast cancer recurrence and death for patients receiving adjuvant endocrine therapy", *CMAJ* 2010; 182: 1857-62.

Adlercreutz, H. "Lignans and human health", *Crit Rev Clin Lab Sci* 2007; 44: 483-525.

Mason, J.K. et L.U. Thompson. "Flaxseed and its lignan and oil components: can they play a role in reducing the risk of and improving the treatment of breast cancer?", *Appl Physiol Nutr Metab* 2014; 39: 663-78.

McCann, S.E. et coll. "Dietary lignan intakes in relation to survival among women with breast cancer: The Western New York Exposures and Breast Cancer (WEB) Study", *Breast Cancer Res Treat* 2010; 122: 229-35.

Lowcock, E.C. et coll. "Consumption of flaxseed, a rich source of lignans, is associated with reduced breast cancer risk", *Cancer Causes Control* 2013; 24: 813-6.

Buck, K. et coll. "Meta-analyses of lignans and enterolignans in relation to breast cancer risk", *Am J Clin Nutr* 2010; 92: 141-153.

## Chapter 9

Aggarwal, B.B. et coll. "Potential of spice-derived phytochemicals for cancer prevention", *Planta Med* 2008; 74: 1560-9.

Gupta, S.C. et coll. "Curcumin, a component of turmeric: from farm to pharmacy", *BioFactors* 2013; 39: 2-13.

Hutchins-Wolfbrandt, A. et A.M. Mistry. "Dietary turmeric potentially reduces the risk of cancer", *Asian Pacific J Cancer Prev* 2011; 12: 3169-3173.

Rastogi, T. et coll. "Cancer incidence rates among South Asians in four geographic regions: India, Singapore, UK and US", *Int J Epidemiol* 2008; 37: 147-60.

Bachmeier, B.E. et coll. "Curcumin downregulates the inflammatory cytokines CXCL1 and -2 in breast cancer cells via NFkappaB", *Carcinogenesis* 2008; 29: 779-89.

Yadav, V.R. et B.B. Aggarwal. "Curcumin: a component of the golden spice, targets multiple angiogenic pathways", *Cancer Biol Ther* 2011; 11: 236-41.

Perkins, S. et coll. "Chemopreventive efficacy and pharmacokinetics of curcumin in the min/+ mouse, a model of familial adenomatous polyposis", *Cancer Epidemiol Biomarkers Prev* 2002; 11: 535-40.

Cheng, A.L. et coll. "Phase I clinical trial of curcumin, a chemopreventive agent, in patients with high-risk or pre-malignant lesions", *Anticancer Res* 2001; 21: 2895-2900.

Sharma, R.A. et coll. "Phase I clinical trial of oral curcumin: biomarkers of systemic activity and compliance", *Clin Cancer Res* 2004; 10: 6847-6854.

Garcea, G. et coll. "Consumption of the putative chemopreventive agent curcumin by cancer patients: assessment of curcumin levels in the colorectum and their pharmacodynamic consequences", *Cancer Epidemiol Biomarkers Prev* 2005; 14: 120-125.

Bayet-Robert, M. et coll. "Phase I dose escalation trial of docetaxel plus curcumin in patients with advanced and metastatic breast cancer", *Cancer Biol Ther* 2010; 9: 8-14.

Dhillon, N. et coll. "Phase II trial of curcumin in patients with advanced pancreatic cancer", *Clin Cancer Res* 2008; 14: 4491-9.

Shoba, G. et coll. "Influence of piperine on the pharmacokinetics of curcumin in animals and human volunteers", *Planta Med* 1998; 64: 353-6.

Dudhatra, G.B. et coll. "A comprehensive review on pharmacotherapeutics of herbal bioenhancers", *Scientific World J* 2012; 2012: 637953.

Cruz-Correa, M. et coll. "Combination treatment with curcumin and quercetin of adenomas in familial adenomatous polyposis", *Clin Gastroenterol Hepatol* 2006; 4: 1035-8.

Kaefer, C.M. et J.A. Milner. "The role of herbs and spices in cancer prevention", *J Nutr Biochem* 2008; 19: 347-61.

Johnson, J.J. "Carnosol: a promising anti-cancer and anti-inflammatory agent", *Cancer Lett* 2011; 305: 1-7.

Shukla, S. et S. Gupta. "Apigenin: a promising molecule for cancer prevention", *Pharm Res* 2010; 27: 962-78.

Lamy, S. et coll. "The dietary flavones apigenin and luteolin impair smooth muscle cell migration and VEGF expression through inhibition of PDGFR-beta phosphorylation", *Cancer Prev Res* 2008; 1: 452-9.

Gates, M.A. et coll. "Flavonoid intake and ovarian cancer risk in a population-based case-control study", *Int J Cancer* 2009; 124: 1918-25.

Meyer, H. et coll. "Bioavailability of apigenin from apiin-rich parsley in humans", *Ann Nutr Metab* 2006; 50: 167-72.

## Chapter 10

Mitscher, L.A. et V. Dolby. *The Green Tea Book: China's Fountain of Youth*, Garden City Park (NY), Avery, 1998, 186 pages.

Rosen, D. *The Book of Green Tea*, North Adams (MA), Storey Publishing, 1998, 160 pages.

Yang, C.S. et coll. "Cancer prevention by tea: animal studies, molecular mechanisms and human relevance", *Nat Rev Cancer* 2009; 9: 429-39.

Singh, B.N. et coll. "Green tea catechin, epigallocatechin-3-gallate (EGCG): mechanisms, perspectives and clinical applications", *Biochem Pharmacol* 2011; 82: 1807-21.

Béliveau, R. et D. Gingras. "Green tea: prevention and treatment of cancer by nutraceuticals", *Lancet* 2004; 364: 1021-1022.

Demeule, M. et coll. "Green tea catechins as novel antitumor and antiangiogenic compounds", *Curr Med Chem Anti-Cancer Agents* 2002; 2: 441-63.

Yuan, J.M. "Cancer prevention by green tea: evidence from epidemiologic studies", *Am J Clin Nutr* 2013; 98: 1676S-1681S.

Yang, G. et coll. "Prospective cohort study of green tea consumption and colorectal cancer risk in women", *Cancer Epidemiol Biomarkers Prev* 2007; 6: 1219-23.

Ide, R. et coll. "A prospective study of green tea consumption and oral cancer incidence in Japan", *Ann Epidemiol* 2007; 17: 821-6.

Kurahashi, N. et coll. "Green tea consumption and prostate cancer risk in Japanese men: a prospective study", *Am J Epidemiol* 2008; 167: 71-7.

Henning, S.M. "Randomized clinical trial of brewed green and black tea in men with prostate cancer prior to prostatectomy", *Prostate* 2015; 75: 550-9.

Tang, N. et coll. "Green tea, black tea consumption and risk of lung cancer: a meta-analysis", *Lung Cancer* 2009; 65: 274-83.

Kurahashi, N. et coll. "Green tea consumption and prostate cancer risk in Japanese men: a prospective study", *Am J Epidemiol* 2008; 167: 71-7.

Zhang, M. et coll. "Green tea and the prevention of breast cancer: a case-control study in Southeast China", *Carcinogenesis* 2007; 28: 1074-8.

Nechuta, S. et coll. "Prospective cohort study of tea consumption and risk of digestive system cancers: results from the Shanghai Women's Health Study", *Am J Clin Nutr* 2012; 96: 1056-63.

Yuan, J.M. "Urinary biomarkers of tea polyphenols and risk of colorectal cancer in the Shanghai Cohort Study", *Int J Cancer* 2007; 120: 1344-50.

Gupta, S. et coll. "Inhibition of prostate carcinogenesis in TRAMP mice by oral infusion of green tea polyphenols", *Proc Natl Acad Sci USA* 2001; 98: 10350-5.

Cao, Y. et R. Cao. "Angiogenesis inhibited by drinking tea", *Nature* 1999; 398: 381.

Lamy, S. et coll. "Green tea catechins inhibit vascular endothelial growth factor receptor phosphorylation", *Cancer Res* 2002; 62: 381-385.

**Chapter 11**

Wang, C.H. et coll. "Cranberry-containing products for prevention of urinary tract infections in susceptible populations: a systematic review and meta-analysis of randomized controlled trials", *Arch Intern Med* 2012; 172: 988-996.

Fung, T.T. et coll. "Intake of specific fruits and vegetables in relation to risk of estrogen receptor-negative breast cancer among postmenopausal women", *Breast Cancer Res Treat* 2013; 138: 925-30.

Hannum, S.M. "Potential impact of strawberries on human health: a review of the science", *Crit Rev Food Sci Nutr* 2004; 44: 1-17.

Carlton, P.S. et coll. "Inhibition of N-nitrosomethylbenzylamine-induced tumorigenesis in the rat esophagus by dietary freeze-dried strawberries", *Carcinogenesis* 2001; 22: 441-446.

Chen, T. et coll. "Randomized phase II trial of lyophilized strawberries in patients with dysplastic precancerous lesions of the esophagus", *Cancer Prev Res* 2012; 5: 41-50.

Wood, W. et coll. "Inhibition of the mutagenicity of bay-region diol epoxides of polycyclic aromatic hydrocarbons by naturally occurring plant phenols: exceptional activity of ellagic acid", *Proc Natl Acad Sci USA* 1982; 79: 5513-5517.

Labrecque, L. et coll. "Combined inhibition of PDGF and VEGF receptors by ellagic acid, a dietary-derived phenolic compound", *Carcinogenesis* 2005; 26: 821-826.

Kong, J.M. et coll. "Analysis and biological activities of anthocyanins", *Phytochemistry* 2003; 64: 923-933.

Lamy, S. et coll. "Delphinidin, a dietary anthocyanidin, inhibits vascular endothelial growth factor receptor-2 phosphorylation", *Carcinogenesis* 2006; 27: 989-96.

Wang, L.S. et coll. "A phase Ib study of the effects of black raspberries on rectal polyps in patients with familial adenomatous polyposis", *Cancer Prev Res* 2014; 7: 666-74.

Rasmussen, S.E. et coll. "Dietary proanthocyanidins: Occurrence, dietary intake, bioavailability, and protection against cardiovascular disease", *Mol Nutr Food Res* 2005; 49: 159-174.

Rossi, M. et coll. "Flavonoids, proanthocyanidins, and cancer risk: a network of case-control studies from Italy", *Nutr Cancer* 2010; 62: 871-877.

Rossi, M. et coll. "Flavonoids, proanthocyanidins, and the risk of stomach cancer", *Cancer Causes Control* 2010; 21: 1597-1604.

Wang, Y. et coll. "Dietary flavonoid and proanthocyanidin intakes and prostate cancer risk in a prospective cohort of US men", *Am J Epidemiol* 2014; 179: 974-86.

**Chapter 12**

Allport, S. *The Queen of Fats: Why Omega-3s Were Removed from the Western Diet and What We Can Do to Replace Them*, Oakland (CA), University of California Press, 2008, 232 pages.

Kris-Etherton, P.M. et coll. "Fish consumption, fish oil, omega-3 fatty acids, and cardiovascular disease", *Circulation* 2002; 106: 2747.

Chan, J.K. et coll. "Effect of dietary alpha-linolenic acid and its ratio to linoleic acid on platelet and plasma fatty acids and thrombogenesis", *Lipids* 1993; 28: 811-7.

De Lorgeril, M. et P. Salen. "New insights into the health effects of dietary saturated and omega-6 and omega-3 polyunsaturated fatty acids", *BMC Med* 2012; 10: 50.

Abel, S. et coll. "Dietary PUFA and cancer", *Proc Nutr Soc* 2014; 73: 361-7.

Mitrou, P.N. et coll. "Mediterranean dietary pattern and prediction of all-cause mortality in a US population: results from the NIH-AARP Diet and Health Study", *Arch Intern Med* 2007; 167: 2461-8.

Filomeno, M. et coll. "Mediterranean diet and risk of endometrial cancer: a pooled analysis of three Italian case-control studies", *Br J Cancer* 2015; 112: 1816.

LeGendre, O. et coll. "Oleocanthal rapidly and selectively induces cancer cell death via lysosomal membrane permeabilization (LMP)", *Mol Cell Oncol* DOI: 10.1080/23723556.2015.1006077.

Lamy, S. et coll. "Olive oil compounds inhibit vascular endothelial growth factor receptor-2 phosphorylation", *Exp Cell Res* 2014; 322: 89-98.

Beauchamp, G.K. et coll. "Phytochemistry: ibuprofen-like activity in extra-virgin olive oil", *Nature* 2005; 437: 45-6.

Peyrot des Gachons, C. et coll. "Unusual pungency from extra-virgin olive oil is attributable to restricted spatial expression of the receptor of oleocanthal", *J Neurosci* 2011; 31: 999-1009.

Uauy, R. et coll. "Essential fatty acids in visual and brain development", *Lipids* 2001; 36: 885-95.

Mozaffarian, D. et J.H. Wu. "(n-3) fatty acids and cardiovascular health: are effects of EPA and DHA shared or complementary?", *J Nutr* 2012; 142: 614S-625S.

Calder, P.C. "Marine omega-3 fatty acids and inflammatory processes: Effects, mechanisms and clinical relevance", *Biochim Biophys Acta* 2015; 1851: 469-484.

Dyerberg, J. et coll. "Fatty acid composition of the plasma lipids in Greenland Eskimos", *Am J Clin Nutr* 1975; 28: 958-66.

Albert, C.M. et coll. "Fish consumption and risk of sudden cardiac death", *JAMA* 1998; 279: 23-8.

Bao, Y. et coll. "Association of nut consumption with total and cause-specific mortality", *N Engl J Med* 2013; 369: 2001-11.

Guasch-Ferré, M. et coll. "Frequency of nut consumption and mortality risk in the PREDIMED nutrition intervention trial", *BMC Med* 2013; 11: 164.

Luu, H.N. et coll. "Prospective evaluation of the association of nut/peanut consumption with total and cause-specific mortality", *JAMA Intern Med* 2015; 175: 755-66.

Grosso, G. et coll. "Nut consumption on all-cause, cardiovascular, and cancer mortality risk: a systematic review and meta-analysis of epidemiologic studies", *Am J Clin Nutr* 2015; 101: 783-93.

Gerber, M. "Omega-3 fatty acids and cancers: a systematic update review of epidemiological studies", *Br J Nutr* 2012; 107: S228-39.

Larsson, S.C. et coll. "Dietary long-chain n-3 fatty acids for the prevention of cancer: a review of potential mechanisms", *Am J Clin Nutr* 2004; 79: 935-945.

Torfadottir, J.E. et coll. "Consumption of fish products across the lifespan and prostate cancer risk", *PLoS One* 2013; 8: e59799.

Hall, M.N. et coll. "A 22-year prospective study of fish, n-3 fatty acid intake, and colorectal cancer risk in men", *Cancer Epidemiol Biomarkers Prev* 2008; 17: 1136-43.

Zheng, J.S. et coll. "Intake of fish and marine n-3 polyunsaturated fatty acids and risk of breast cancer: meta-analysis of data from 21 independent prospective cohort studies", *BMJ* 2013; 346: f3706.

Sawada, N. et coll. "Consumption of n-3 fatty acids and fish reduces risk of hepatocellular carcinoma", *Gastroenterology* 2012; 142: 1468-75.

Epstein, M.M. "Dietary fatty acid intake and prostate cancer survival in Örebro County, Sweden", *Am J Epidemiol* 2012; 176: 240-52.

Khankari, N.K. "Dietary intake of fish, polyunsaturated fatty acids, and survival after breast cancer: A population-based follow-up study on Long Island, New York", *Cancer* 2015 Mar 24. doi: 10.1002/cncr.29329.

Szymanski, K.M. "Fish consumption and prostate cancer risk: a review and meta-analysis", *Am J Clin Nutr* 2010; 92: 1223-33.

Brasky, T.M. et coll. "Long-chain Ω-3 fatty acid intake and endometrial cancer risk in the Women's Health Initiative", *Am J Clin Nutr* 2015; 101: 824-34.

## Chapter 13

Wertz, K. et coll. "Lycopene: modes of action to promote prostate health", *Arch Biochem Biophys* 2004; 430: 127-134.

Shi, J. et M. Le Maguer. "Lycopene in tomatoes: chemical and physical properties affected by food processing", *Crit Rev Food Sci Nutr* 2000; 40: 1-42.

Unlu, N.Z. et coll. "Lycopene from heat-induced cis-isomer-rich tomato sauce is more bioavailable than from all-trans-rich tomato sauce in human subjects", *Br J Nutr* 2007; 98: 140-6.

Giovannucci, E. "Tomatoes, tomato-based products, lycopene, and cancer: review of the epidemiologic literature", *J Natl Cancer Inst* 1999; 91: 317-31.

Giovannucci, E. et coll. "A prospective study of tomato products, lycopene, and prostate cancer risk", *J Natl Cancer Inst* 2002; 94: 391-8.

Wu, K. et coll. "Plasma and dietary carotenoids, and the risk of prostate cancer: a nested case-control study", *Cancer Epidemiol Biomarkers Prev* 2004; 13: 260-9.

Campbell, J.K. et coll. "Tomato phytochemicals and prostate cancer risk", *J Nutr* 2004; 134: 3486S-3492S.

Sharoni, Y. et coll. "The role of lycopene and its derivatives in the regulation of transcription systems: implications for cancer prevention", *Am J Clin Nutr* 2012; 96: 1173S-8S.

Khachik, F. et coll. "Chemistry, distribution, and metabolism of tomato carotenoids and their impact on human health", *Exp Biol Med* 2002; 227: 845-51.

Ho, W.J. et coll. "Antioxidant micronutrients and the risk of renal cell carcinoma in the Women's Health Initiative cohort", *Cancer* 2015; 121: 580-8.

Giovannucci, E. et coll. "Intake of carotenoids and retinol in relation to risk of prostate cancer", *J Natl Cancer Inst* 1995; 87: 1767-76.

Eliassen, A.H. et coll. "Circulating carotenoids and risk of breast cancer: pooled analysis of eight prospective studies", *J Natl Cancer Inst* 2012; 104: 1905-16.

Zhang, X. et coll. "Carotenoid intakes and risk of breast cancer defined by estrogen receptor and progesterone receptor status: a pooled analysis

of 18 prospective cohort studies", *Am J Clin Nutr* 2012; 95: 713-25.

Rizwan, M. et coll. "Tomato paste rich in lycopene protects against cutaneous photodamage in humans in vivo: a randomized controlled trial", *Br J Dermatol* 2011; 164: 154-162.

Ross, A.B. et coll. "Lycopene bioavailability and metabolism in humans: an accelerator mass spectrometry study", *Am J Clin Nutr* 2011; 93: 1263-1273.

## Chapter 14

Wu, G.A. et coll. "Sequencing of diverse mandarin, pummelo and orange genomes reveals complex history of admixture during citrus domestication", *Nat Biotechnol* 2014; 32: 656-62.

Gmitter, F.G. et X. Hu. "The possible role of Yunnan, China, in the origin of contemporary citrus species (*Rutaceae*)", *Economic Botany* 1990; 44: 267-277.

Arias, B.A. et L. Ramon-Laca. "Pharmacological properties of citrus and their ancient and medieval uses in the Mediterranean region", *J Ethnopharm* 2005; 97: 89-95.

Manthey, J.A. et coll. "Biological properties of citrus flavonoids pertaining to cancer and inflammation", *Curr Med Chem* 2001; 8: 135-153.

Crowell, P.L. "Prevention and therapy of cancer by dietary monoterpenes", *J Nutr* 1999; 129: 775S-778S.

Gonzalez, C.A. et coll. "Fruit and vegetable intake and the risk of gastric adenocarcinoma: a reanalysis of the European Prospective Investigation into Cancer and Nutrition (EPIC-EURGAST) study after a longer follow-up", *Int J Cancer* 2012; 131: 2910-9.

Steevens, J. et coll. "Vegetables and fruits consumption and risk of esophageal and gastric cancer subtypes in the Netherlands Cohort Study", *Int J Cancer* 2011; 129: 2681-93.

Maserejian, N.N. et coll. "Prospective study of fruits and vegetables and risk of oral premalignant lesions in men", *Am J Epidemiol* 2006; 164: 556-66.

Li, W.Q. et coll. "Citrus consumption and cancer incidence: the Ohsaki cohort study", *Int J Cancer* 2010; 127: 1913-22.

Kwan, M.L. et coll. "Food consumption by children and the risk of childhood acute leukemia", *Am J Epidemiol* 2004; 160: 1098-107.

Bailey, D.G. et coll. "Grapefruit juice-drug interactions", *Br J Clin Pharmacol* 1998; 46: 101-110.

## Chapter 15

Aradhya, M. et coll. "Genetic structure, differentiation, and phylogeny of the genus vitis: implications for genetic conservation", *Acta Hortic (ISHS)* 2008; 799: 43-49.

McGovern, P.E. et coll. "Neolithic resinated wine", *Nature* 1996; 381: 480-481.

This, P. et coll. "Historical origins and genetic diversity of wine grapes", *Trends Genet* 2006; 22: 511-9.

St-Leger, A.S. et coll. "Factors associated with cardiac mortality in developed countries with particular reference to the consumption of wine", *Lancet* 1979; 1: 1017-1020.

Renaud, S. et M. de Lorgeril. "Wine, alcohol, platelets, and the French paradox for coronary heart disease", *Lancet* 1992; 339: 1523-1526.

De Lorgeril, M. et coll. "Wine drinking and risks of cardiovascular complications after recent acute myocardial infarction", *Circulation* 2002; 106: 1465-9.

Di Castelnuovo, A. et coll. "Meta-analysis of wine and beer consumption in relation to vascular risk", *Circulation* 2002; 105: 2836-2844.

Di Castelnuovo, A. et coll. "Alcohol dosing and total mortality in men and women: an updated meta-analysis of 34 prospective studies", *Arch Intern Med* 2006; 166: 2437-45.

Szmitko, P.E. et S. Verma. "Red wine and your heart" *Circulation* 2005; 111: e10-e11.

Gronbaek, M. et coll. "Type of alcohol consumed and mortality from all causes, coronary heart disease, and cancer", *Ann Intern Med* 2000; 133: 411-419.

Klatsky, A.L. et coll. "Wine, liquor, beer, and mortality", *Am J Epidemiol* 2003; 158: 585-595.

Renaud, S.C. et coll. "Wine, beer, and mortality in middle-aged men from eastern France", *Arch Intern Med* 1999; 159: 1865-1870.

Frankel, E.N. et coll. "Inhibition of oxidation of human low-density lipoprotein by phenolic substances in red wine", *Lancet* 1993; 341: 454-7.

Chiva-Blanch, G. et coll. "Effects of red wine polyphenols and alcohol on glucose metabolism and the lipid profile: a randomized clinical trial", *Clin Nutr* 2013; 32: 200-6.

German, J.B. et R.L. Walzem. "The health benefits of wine", *Annu Rev Nutr* 2000; 20: 561-593.

Langcake, P. et coll. "Production of resveratrol by *Vitis vinifera* and other members of *Vitaceae* as a response to infection or injury", *Physiol Plant Pathol* 1976; 9: 77-86.

Baan, R. et coll. "Carcinogenicity of alcoholic beverages", *Lancet Oncol* 2007; 8: 292-3.

Salaspuro, V. et M. Salaspuro. "Synergistic effect of alcohol drinking and smoking on in vivo acetaldehyde concentration in saliva", *Int J Cancer* 2004; 111: 480-3.

Castellsagué, X. et coll. "The role of type of tobacco and type of alcoholic beverage in oral carcinogenesis", *Int J Cancer* 2004; 108: 741-9.

Chao, C. "Associations between beer, wine, and liquor consumption and lung cancer risk: a meta-analysis", *Cancer Epidemiol Biomarkers Prev* 2007; 16: 2436-47.

Benedetti, A. et coll. "Lifetime consumption of alcoholic beverages and risk of 13 types of cancer in men: results from a case-control study in Montreal", *Cancer Detect Prev* 2009; 32: 352-62.

Allen, N.E. et coll. "Moderate alcohol intake and cancer incidence in women", *J Natl Cancer Inst* 2009; 101: 296-305.

Jang, M. et coll. "Cancer chemopreventive activity of resveratrol, a natural product derived from grapes", *Science* 1997; 275: 218-20.

Kraft, T.E. et coll. "Fighting cancer with red wine? Molecular mechanisms of resveratrol", *Crit Rev Food Sci Nutr* 2009; 49: 782-99.

Patel, K.R. et coll. "Sulfate metabolites provide an intracellular pool for resveratrol generation and induce autophagy with senescence", *Sci Transl Med* 2013; 5: 205ra133.

Fontana, L. et L. Partridge. "Promoting health and longevity through diet: from model organisms to humans", *Cell* 2015; 161: 106-18.

Wood, J.G. et coll. "Sirtuin activators mimic caloric restriction and delay ageing in metazoans", *Nature* 2004; 430: 686-689.

Sajish, M. et P. Schimmel. "A human tRNA synthetase is a potent PARP1-activating effector target for resveratrol", *Nature* 2015; 519: 370-3.

## Chapter 16

Burkitt, D.P. "Epidemiology of cancer of the colon and rectum", *Cancer* 1971; 28: 3-13.

Bradbury, K.E. et coll. "Fruit, vegetable, and fiber intake in relation to cancer risk: findings from the European Prospective Investigation into Cancer and Nutrition (EPIC)", *Am J Clin Nutr* 2014; 100: 394S-8S.

Aune, D. et coll. "Dietary fibre, whole grains, and risk of colorectal cancer: systematic review and dose-response meta-analysis of prospective studies", *BMJ* 2011; 343: d6617.

Huang, T. et coll. "Consumption of whole grains and cereal fiber and total and cause-specific mortality: prospective analysis of 367,442 individuals", *BMC Med* 2015; 13: 59.

Louis, P. et coll. "The gut microbiota, bacterial metabolites and colorectal cancer", *Nat Rev Microbiol* 2014; 12: 661-72.

Schwabe, R.F. et C. Jobin. "The microbiome and cancer", *Nat Rev Cancer* 2013; 13: 800-12.

Ahn, J. et coll. "Human gut microbiome and risk for colorectal cancer", *J Natl Cancer Inst* 2013; 105: 1907-11.

Kostic, A.D. et coll. "*Fusobacterium nucleatum* potentiates intestinal tumorigenesis and modulates the tumor-immune microenvironment", *Cell Host Microbe* 2013; 14: 207-15.

Yoshimoto, S. et coll. "Obesity-induced gut microbial metabolite promotes liver cancer through senescence secretome", *Nature* 2013; 499: 97-101.

Turnbaugh, P.J. et coll. "A core gut microbiome in obese and lean twins", *Nature* 2009; 457: 480-4.

Everard, A. et P.D. Cani. "Diabetes, obesity and gut microbiota", *Best Pract Res Clin Gastroenterol* 2013; 27: 73-83.

Sampson, T.R. et S.K. Mazmanian. "Control of brain development, function, and behavior by the microbiome", *Cell Host Microbe* 2015; 17: 565-576.

O'Keefe, S.J. et coll. "Fat, fibre and cancer risk in African Americans and rural Africans", *Nature Commun* 2015; 6: 6342.

Chassaing, B. et coll. "Dietary emulsifiers impact the mouse gut microbiota promoting colitis and metabolic syndrome", *Nature* 2015; 519: 92-6.

Suez, J. et coll. "Artificial sweeteners induce glucose intolerance by altering the gut microbiota", *Nature* 2014; 514: 181-6.

David, L.A. et coll. "Diet rapidly and reproducibly alters the human gut microbiome", *Nature* 2014; 505: 559-63.

Valverde, M.E. et coll. "Edible mushrooms: improving human health and promoting quality life", *Int J Microbiol* 2015; 2015: 376387.

Ikekawa, T. "Beneficial effects of edible and medicinal mushrooms on health care", *Int J Med Mushrooms* 2001; 3: 291-298.

Hara, M. et coll. "Cruciferous vegetables, mushrooms, and gastrointestinal cancer risks in a multicenter, hospital-based case-control study in Japan", *Nutr Cancer* 2003; 46: 138-47.

Li, J. et coll. "Dietary mushroom intake may reduce the risk of breast cancer: evidence from a meta-analysis of observational studies", *PLoS One* 2014; 9: e93437.

Schwartz, B. et Y. Hadar. "Possible mechanisms of action of mushroom-derived glucans on inflammatory bowel disease and associated cancer", *Ann Transl Med* 2014; 2: 19.

Ina, K. et coll. "The use of lentinan for treating gastric cancer", *Anticancer Agents Med Chem* 2013; 13: 681-8.

Maehara, Y. et coll. "Biological mechanism and clinical effect of protein-bound polysaccharide K (KRESTIN(®)): review of development and future perspectives", *Surg Today* 2012; 42: 8-28.

Chen, S. et coll. "Anti-aromatase activity of phytochemicals in white button mushrooms (*Agaricus bisporus*)", *Cancer Res* 2006; 66: 12026-34.

Lee, A.H. et coll. "Mushroom intake and risk of epithelial ovarian cancer in southern Chinese women", *Int J Gynecol Cancer* 2013; 23: 1400-5.

Twardowski, P. et coll. "A phase I trial of mushroom powder in patients with biochemically recurrent prostate cancer: Roles of cytokines and myeloid-derived suppressor cells for *Agaricus bisporus*-induced prostate-specific antigen responses", *Cancer* 2015 May 18; doi: 10.1002/cncr.29421.

Hehemann, J.H. et coll. "Transfer of carbohydrate-active enzymes from marine bacteria to Japanese gut microbiota", *Nature* 2010; 464: 908-12.

Skibola, C.F. et coll. "Brown kelp modulates endocrine hormones in female sprague-dawley rats and in human luteinized granulosa cells", *J Nutr* 2005; 135: 296-300.

Teas, J. et coll. "Dietary seaweed modifies estrogen and phytoestrogen metabolism in healthy postmenopausal women", *J Nutr* 2009; 139: 939-44.

Yang, Y.J. et coll. "A case-control study on seaweed consumption and the risk of breast cancer", *Br J Nutr* 2010; 103: 1345-53.

Hoshiyama, Y. et coll. "A case-control study of colorectal cancer and its relation to diet, cigarettes, and alcohol consumption in Saitama Prefecture, Japan", *Tohoku J Exp Med* 1993; 171: 153-65.

Senthilkumar, K. et S.K. Kim. "Anticancer effects of fucoidan", *Adv Food Nutr Res* 2014; 72: 195-213.

Rengarajan, T. et coll. "Cancer preventive efficacy of marine carotenoid fucoxanthin: cell cycle arrest and apoptosis", *Nutrients* 2013; 5: 4978-89.

Kotake-Nara, E. et coll. "Neoxanthin and fucoxanthin induce apoptosis in PC-3 human prostate cancer cells", *Cancer Lett* 2005; 220: 75-84.

Sreekumar, S. et coll. "Pomegranate fruit as a rich source of biologically active compounds", *Biomed Res Int* 2014; 2014: 686921.

Khan, N. et coll. "Oral consumption of pomegranate fruit extract inhibits growth and progression of primary lung tumors in mice", *Cancer Res* 2007; 67: 3475-3482.

Malik, A. et coll. "Pomegranate fruit juice for chemoprevention and chemotherapy of prostate cancer", *Proc Natl Acad Sci USA* 2005; 102: 14813-14818.

Pantuck, A.J. et coll. "Phase II study of pomegranate juice for men with rising prostate-specific antigen following surgery or radiation for prostate cancer", *Clin Cancer Res* 2006; 12: 4018-4026.

Thomas, R. et coll. "A double-blind, placebo-controlled randomised trial evaluating the effect of a polyphenol-rich whole food supplement on PSA progression in men with prostate cancer – the U.K. NCRN Pomi-T study", *Prostate Cancer Prostatic Dis* 2014; 17: 180-6.

Andres-Lacueva, C. et coll. "Phenolic compounds: chemistry and occurrence in fruits and vegetables", dans de la Rosa, L.A., E. Alvarez-Parrilla et G.A. Gonzalez-Aguilar, dirs. *Fruit and Vegetable Phytochemicals: Chemistry, Nutritional Value and Stability*, Ames (IA), Wiley-Blackwell, 2009, 384 pages.

Feskanich, D. et coll. "Prospective study of fruit and vegetable consumption and risk of lung cancer among men and women", *J Natl Cancer Inst* 2000; 92: 1812-23.

Freedman, N.D. et coll. "Fruit and vegetable intake and head and neck cancer risk in a large United States prospective cohort study", *Int J Cancer* 2008; 122: 2330-6.

Noratto, G. et coll. "Identifying peach and plum polyphenols with chemopreventive potential against estrogen-independent breast cancer cells", *J Agric Food Chem* 2009; 57: 5219-26.

Noratto, G. et coll. "Polyphenolics from peach (*Prunus persica* var. Rich Lady) inhibit tumor growth and metastasis of MDA-MB-435 breast cancer cells in vivo", *J Nutr Biochem* 2014; 25: 796-800.

Fung, T.T. et coll. "Intake of specific fruits and vegetables in relation to risk of estrogen receptor-negative breast cancer among postmenopausal women", *Breast Cancer Res Treat* 2013; 138: 925-30.

Nkondjock, A. "Coffee consumption and the risk of cancer: an overview", *Cancer Lett* 2009; 277: 121-5.

Yu, X. et coll. "Coffee consumption and risk of cancers: a meta-analysis of cohort studies", *BMC Cancer* 2011; 11: 96.

Li, J. et coll. "Coffee consumption modifies risk of estrogen-receptor negative breast cancer", *Breast Cancer Research* 2011; 13: R49.

Bamia, C. et coll. "Coffee, tea and decaffeinated coffee in relation to hepatocellular carcinoma in a European population: multicentre, prospective cohort study", *Int. J. Cancer* 2015; 136: 1899-908.

Rosendahl, A.H. et coll. "Caffeine and caffeic acid inhibit growth and modify estrogen receptor and insulin-like growth factor I receptor levels in human breast cancer", *Clin Cancer Res* 2015; 21: 1877-87.

Hurst, W. J. et coll. "Cacao usage by the earliest Maya civilization", *Nature* 2002; 418: 289-290.

Dillinger, T.L. et coll. "Food of the gods: cure for humanity? A cultural history of the medicinal and ritual use of chocolate", *J Nutr* 2000; 130: 2057S-2072S.

Kim, J. et coll. "Cocoa phytochemicals: recent advances in molecular mechanisms on health", *Crit Rev Food Sci Nutr* 2014; 54: 1458-72.

Buijsse, B. et coll. "Cocoa intake, blood pressure, and cardiovascular mortality: the Zutphen Elderly Study", *Arch Intern Med* 2006; 166: 411-417.

Lewis, J.R, et coll. "Habitual chocolate intake and vascular disease: a prospective study of clinical outcomes in older women", *Arch Intern Med* 2010; 170: 1857-1858.

di Giuseppe, R. et coll. "Regular consumption of dark chocolate is associated with low serum concentrations of C-reactive protein in a healthy Italian population", *J Nutr* 2008; 138: 1939-45.

Schroeter, H. et coll. "(-)-Epicatechin mediates beneficial effects of flavanol-rich cocoa on vascular function in humans", *Proc Natl Acad Sci USA* 2006; 103: 1024-9.

Serafini, M. et coll. "Plasma antioxidants from chocolate", *Nature* 2003; 424: 1013.

Mastroiacovo, D. et coll. "Cocoa flavanol consumption improves cognitive function, blood pressure control, and metabolic profile in elderly subjects: the Cocoa, Cognition, and Aging (CoCoA) Study – a randomized controlled trial", *Am J Clin Nutr* 2015; 101: 538-48.

Messerli, F.H. "Chocolate consumption, cognitive function, and Nobel laureates", *N Engl J Med* 2012; 367: 1562-4.

Wang, Y. et coll. "Dietary flavonoid and proanthocyanidin intakes and prostate cancer risk in a prospective cohort of US men", *Am J Epidemiol* 2014; 179: 974-86.

Cutler, G.J. et coll. "Dietary flavonoid intake and risk of cancer in postmenopausal women: the Iowa Women's Health Study", *Int J Cancer* 2008; 123: 664-71.

Zamora-Ros, R. et coll. "Dietary flavonoid, lignan and antioxidant capacity and risk of hepatocellular carcinoma in the European prospective investigation into cancer and nutrition study", *Int J Cancer* 2013; 133: 2429-43.

Zamora-Ros, R. et coll. "Flavonoid and lignan intake in relation to bladder cancer risk in the

European Prospective Investigation into Cancer and Nutrition (EPIC) study", *Br J Cancer* 2014; 111: 1870-80.

Cassidy, A. et coll. "Intake of dietary flavonoids and risk of epithelial ovarian cancer", *Am J Clin Nutr* 2014; 100: 1344-51.

Spadafranca, A. et coll. "Effect of dark chocolate on plasma epicatechin levels, DNA resistance to oxidative stress and total antioxidant activity in healthy subjects", *Br J Nutr* 2010; 103: 1008-14.

Kenny, T.P. et coll. "Cocoa procyanidins inhibit proliferation and angiogenic signals in human dermal microvascular endothelial cells following stimulation by low-level H2O2", *Exp Biol Med* 2004; 229: 765-771.

Etxeberria, U. et coll. "Impact of polyphenols and polyphenol-rich dietary sources on gut microbiota composition", *J Agric Food Chem* 2013; 61: 9517-33.

Tzounis, X. et coll. "Prebiotic evaluation of cocoa-derived flavanols in healthy humans by using a randomized, controlled, double-blind, crossover intervention study", *Am J Clin Nutr* 2011; 93: 62-72.

Moore, M. et J. Finley. "The precise reason for the health benefits of dark chocolate: mystery solved", 247th Meeting of the American Chemical Society, Dallas, 18 mars 2014.

**Chapter 17**

Hecht, S.S. "Tobacco Smoke Carcinogens and Lung Cancer", *J Natl Cancer Inst* 1999; 91: 1194-1210.

Doll, R. et coll. "Mortality in relation to smoking: 50 years' observations on male British doctors", *BMJ* 2004; 328: 1519.

Fairchild, A.L. et coll. "The renormalization of smoking? E-cigarettes and the tobacco "endgame"", *N Engl J Med* 2014; 370: 293-5.

Grana, R. et coll. "E-cigarettes: a scientific review", *Circulation* 2014; 129: 1972-86.

Arem, H. et coll. "Physical activity and cancer-specific mortality in the NIH-AARP Diet and Health Study cohort", *Int J Cancer* 2014; 135: 423-31.

Schmid, D. et M. Leitzmann. "Television viewing and time spent sedentary in relation to cancer risk: a meta-analysis", *J Natl Cancer Inst* 2014; 106: pii: dju098.

Giovannucci, E.L. "Physical activity as a standard cancer treatment", *J Natl Cancer Inst* 2012; 104: 797-9.

Di Castelnuovo, A. et coll. "Alcohol dosing and total mortality in men and women: an updated meta-analysis of 34 prospective studies", *Arch Intern Med* 2006; 166: 2437-45.

Allen, N.E. et coll. "Moderate alcohol intake and cancer incidence in women", *J Natl Cancer Inst* 2009; 101: 296-305.

Kwan, M.L. et coll. "Alcohol consumption and breast cancer recurrence and survival among women with early-stage breast cancer: The Life After Cancer Epidemiology (LACE) Study", *J Clin Oncol* 2010; 28: 4410-4416.

Green, A.C., G.M. Williams, V. Logan et coll. "Reduced melanoma after regular sunscreen use: randomized control trial follow-up", *J Clin Oncol* 2011; 29: 257-263.

Zhang, M. "Use of tanning beds and incidence of skin cancer", *J Clin Oncol* 2012; 30: 1588-1593.

Joossens, J.V. et coll. "Dietary salt, nitrate and stomach cancer mortality in 24 countries. European Cancer Prevention (ECP) and the INTERSALT Cooperative Research Group", *Int J Epidemiol* 1996; 25: 494-504.

Lampe, J.W. "Spicing up a vegetarian diet: chemopreventive effects of phytochemicals", *Am J Clin Nutr* 2003; 78: 579S-583S.

Macpherson, H. et coll. "Multivitamin-multimineral supplementation and mortality: a meta-analysis of randomized controlled trials", *Am J Clin Nutr* 2013; 97: 437-44.

Bjelakovic, G. et coll. "Antioxidant supplements and mortality", *Curr Opin Clin Nutr Metab Care* 14 novembre 2013.

Giovannucci, E. et coll. "Prospective study of predictors of vitamin D status and cancer incidence and mortality in men", *J Natl Cancer Inst* 2006; 98: 451-459.

Feldman, D. et coll. "The role of Vitamin D in reducing cancer risk and progression", *Nat Rev Cancer* 2014; 14: 342-57.

Williams, S.C.P. "Link between obesity and cancer", *Proc Natl Acad Sci USA* 2013; 110: 8753-54.

Stewart, S.T. et coll. "Forecasting the effects of obesity and smoking on U.S. life expectancy", *N Engl J Med* 2009; 361: 2252-60.

Chan, D.S. et coll. "Red and processed meat and colorectal cancer incidence: meta-analysis of prospective studies", *PLoS One* 2011; 6: e20456.

Sinha, R. et coll. "Meat intake and mortality: a prospective study of over half a million people", *Arch Intern Med* 2009; 169: 562-71.

Khafif, A. et coll. "Quantitation of chemopreventive synergism between (-)-epigallocatechin-3-gallate and curcumin in normal, premalignant and malignant human oral epithelial cells", *Carcinogenesis* 1998; 19: 419-24.

Annabi, B. et coll. "Radiation induced-tubulogenesis in endothelial cells is antagonized by the antiangiogenic properties of green tea polyphenol (-)-epigallocatechin-3-gallate", *Cancer Biol Ther* 2003; 2: 642-649.

Shoba, G. et coll. "Influence of piperine on the pharmacokinetics of curcumin in animals and human volunteers", *Planta Med* 1998; 64: 353-6.

Sehgal, A. et coll. "Combined effects of curcumin and piperine in ameliorating benzo(a)pyrene induced DNA damage", *Food Chem Toxicol* 2011; 49: 3002-6.

E. Toledo et coll., "Mediterranean Diet and Invasive Breast Cancer Risk Among Women at High Cardiovascular Risk in the PREDIMED Trial: A Randomized Clinical Trial", *JAMA Intern Med.*, doi:10.1001/jamainternmed.2015.4838, publié en ligne le 14 septembre 2015.

Kakarala, M. et coll. "Targeting breast stem cells with the cancer preventive compounds curcumin and piperine", *Breast Cancer Res Treat* 2010; 122: 777-85.

Liu, R.H. "Potential synergy of phytochemicals in cancer prevention: mechanism of action", *J Nutr* 2004; 134: 3479S-3485S.

## IMAGE CREDITS

**Michel Rouleau**

31, 35, 39, 44, 48, 50, 68, 70, 78

**Shutterstock**

C1a: Dream79; C1b: iLight photo; C1c: Yasuhiro Amano; C1d: Natu; C1e: James Passale-Poissant; C1f: Francesco83; C1g: Elovich; C1h: Triff; C1i: Holbox; C1j: Sinan Niyazi Kutsal; C1k: Aprilphoto; C4a: Guzel Studio; C4b: Dusan Zidar; C4c: Stockcreations; C4d: Iryna1; 6-7: Gleb Semenjuk; 10: Convit; 11, 71a: Binh Thanh Bui; 12: Alan Bailey; 14: Aila Images; 15: hase4Studios; 16: Alan Poulson Photography; 17: Farley Thurdumond; 18: AJP; 19: KPG_Payless; 20: MickyWiswedel; 22: Wallenrock; 23: Bothy Descin; 25: M. Unal Ozmen; 28: sl_photo; 33: Janez Volmajer; 35, 45, 48, 88: Mitch Chan Groult-Thulmer; 42: Chepko Danil Vitalevich; 46:

Toeytoey; 47, 52: Sebastian Kaulitzki; 49: Umit Erdem; 50: Ljupco Smokovski; 51, 173: Alexander Raths; 56: IngridHS; 58: Ortodox; 59a: Jiang Hongyan; 59b: NataliTerr; 61: Kjersti Joergensen; 62: Petarg; 63a: Stephen Mcsweeny; 63b: Svry; 65: Mega Pixel; 66: Minerva Studio; 69a: Auremar; 69b: Anna Lurye; 71b: Preto Perola; 72: Bikeriderlondon; 74, 94, 110, 111: Africa Studio; 77, 82, 241: Nattika; 79: Valentina Razumova; 81a: Candus Camera; 81b, 153: Laitr Keiows; 83: Zoom Team; 84: James-Susie Aunsel Reysurin-Podewrs; 86: co; Sebastian Kaulitzki; 87: Guru 3D; 90: Liza1979; 91: Tropper2000; 92: Errey Images; 97: Stockcreations; 98: Gayvoronskaya_Yana; 99: Photosync; 100: Ksena2you; 101: Pilipphoto; 102: Nipaporn Panyacharoen; 106: Adriana Nikolova; 109: Pawel Michalowski; 112: Maks Narodenko; 113: MaraZe; 114: Vladimir Volodin; 118: Deeepblue; 120: Cocone; 121: Slonme; 122: Jiri Hera; 124: Sevenke; 126: Sunabesyou; 128: Bonchan; 130: Jose115; 132: Iakov Kalinin; 133: Csaba Deli; 136: Krzysztof Slusarczyk; 138: Jayla Buchan-Pheult; 141, 154: Szefei; 142: Perfect Lazybones; 143: Kenishirotie; 143: Aiken Holt-Klaust; 145: Elena Schweitzer; 148: Cuson; 150: Kai Keisuke; 155: Nishihama; 156a: Shanshan Gao; 156b: MaraZe; 157: Piyato; 160: Sasa Komlen; 163: Alex Staroseltsev; 165: Eye-blink; 166: Nata-Lia; 167: NinaM; 168: Miguel Garcia Saavedra; 169a: ANCH; 169b: JOAT; 174: Doug Nolt; 175: Ewais; 176: Fotyma; 177: Lee Pild; 179: Angel Simon; 180: HLPhoto; 184: Slavica Stajic; 186: Tischenko Irina; 188: Ana Photo; 189: Gargantiopa; 192: Elizaveta Shagliy; 194: Murengstockphoto; 195: Diana Taliun; 196: Svetlana Lukienko; 197: Valentyn Volkov; 200: Stokkete; 205: Mauro Rodrigues; 206: Somchai Som; 211: Wavebreakmedia; 214: Reika; 216: AlenKadr; 219: Yochika photographer; 220: Elena Elisseeva; 223: Ostancov Vladislav; 224: HandmadePictures; 226: Ioannis Pantzi; 228: Natali Zakharova; 229: Davydenko Yuliia; 232: Pio3; 233, 250: Matin; 234: Mustafa Ertugral; 236: Aleksey Sagitov; 237: Lifebrary; 238: Mladen Mitrinovic; 239: Alex Malikov; 241: Charles Coultry; 244: Nenov Brothers Images; 248: Angel Simon; 249b: Alena Hovorkova; 251: Dinesh Picholiya; 253: HLPhoto

# Index